Nutrition for Children

Also of interest from M&K Publishing

Books can be ordered online at: www.mkupdate.co.uk

Pre-Teen and Teenage Pregnancy

ISBN: 978-1-905539-11-6

Inter-professional Approaches to Young Fathers

ISBN: 978-1-905539-29-1

Interpersonal Skills workbook

ISBN: 978-1-905539-37-6

Loss & Grief workbook

ISBN: 978-1-905539-43-7

Nutritional Care of Older People workbook

ISBN: 978-1-905539-05-5

Identification and Treatment of Alcohol Dependency

ISBN: 978-1-905539-16-1

Music makes a difference
A practical guide to developing music with people with learning disabilities

ISBN: 978-1-905539-19-2

Nutrition for Children
A no-nonsense guide for parents

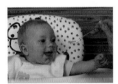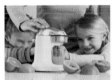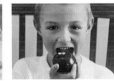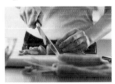

Dr Wyndham Boobier, PhD, MSc, BA

Nutrition for Children

A no-nonsense guide for parents

Dr Wyndham Boobier

ISBN: 978-1-905539-26-0

First published 2008

British Library Catalogue in Publication Data

A catalogue record for this book is available from the British Library

Notice

Clinical practice and medical knowledge constantly evolve. Standard safety precautions must be followed, but, as knowledge is broadened by research, changes in practice, treatment and drug therapy may become necessary or appropriate. Any brands mentioned in this book are as examples only and are not endorsed by the Publisher. Neither the publisher nor the author assume any liability for any injury and/or damage to persons or property arising from this publication.

The Publisher

To contact M&K Publishing write to:
M&K Update Ltd · The Old Bakery · St. John's Street
Keswick · Cumbria CA12 5AS
Tel: 01768 773030 · Fax: 01768 781099
publishing@mkupdate.co.uk
www.mkupdate.co.uk

Designed & typeset by Mary Blood

Printed in England by Freebird Print Management

Contents

List of figures

List of tables

About the Author

Dr Boobier is one of those unusual individuals who has remained at the cutting edge of food science and nutrition through combining his experiences as a university academic and a senior manager in food production. His lecturing on nutritional health throughout the schools of Wales have been highly acclaimed and there is always a keen gathering of schools seeking to use his outstanding communication skills. He holds a Bachelor's degree in Biological Sciences, a Master's degree in Nutritional Biochemistry and a PhD in Functional Food Developments and Selected Heart Disease Risk Factors. He is a Registered Nutritionist, a Fellow of the Royal Society of Health, a Chartered Biologist and a consultant to the baking industry. Dr Boobier has published a number of papers in peer reviewed journals.

As a researcher in the university he is constantly trying to change the structure of foods so that they contain a high level of nutritional quality prior to being presented for consumption by the public. It was the experience gained from meeting the people of Wales and talking about nutrition with individual families that inspired Dr Boobier to write this book. This is a gem of knowledge that has been cooked to perfection for the public's consumption.

Acknowledgements

This book was written with the help of a number of people and I would like to express my appreciation for their valued contributions. To Elaine Farrell for proofreading the manuscript, to Fliss Watts for her attention to detail and valued advice in editing the manuscript.
To my wife and daughter (Morfydd and Emma) who supplied endless cups of coffee and encouragement. Morfydd was instrumental in getting me started and provided feedback as a parent throughout the writing of the book. Finally to the many thousands of people who attended my nutrition and health promotion presentations throughout Wales over the past five years.

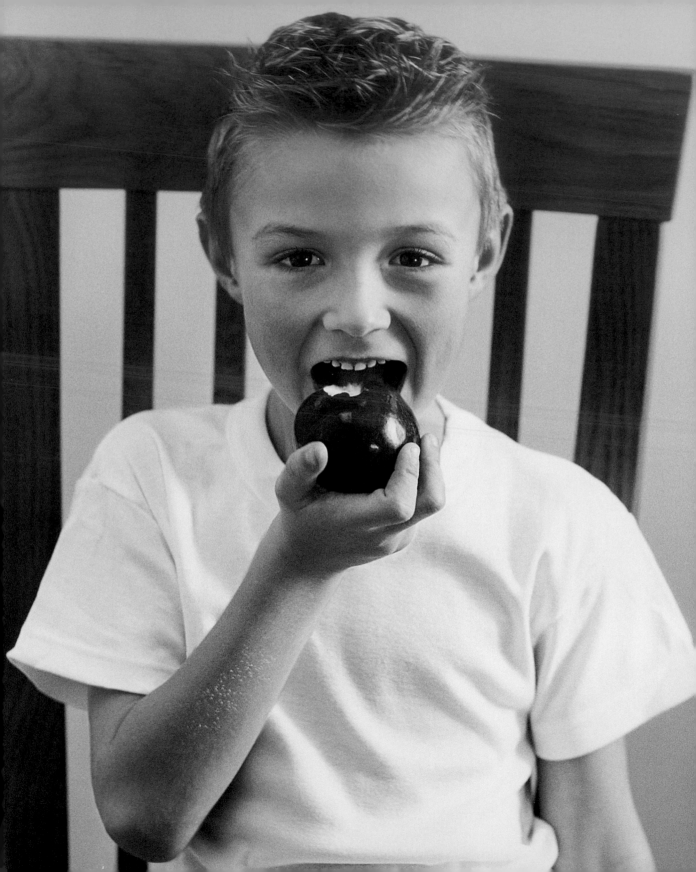

Introduction

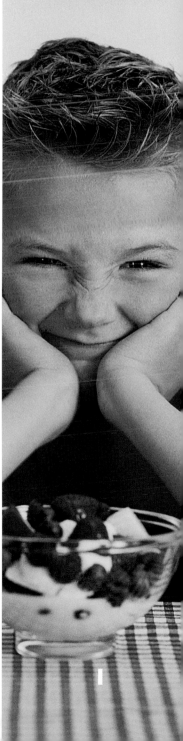

I have often thought how nice it would be to read a book about children's nutrition that was written for parents by a parent. Such a book would be straightforward, easy to understand and would not be full of obscure facts and statistics. So I thought why not write it myself. I'm a father and a nutritionist with a great deal of experience having spent over five years giving lectures on human nutrition and health promotion to parents and children of all ages throughout Wales. This book is the result. I do not claim it to be the most comprehensive 'text' about nutrition, but it is written for parents and carers of children who are truly concerned about their health.

I hope you will find the book useful and enjoyable. Use the book as a reference; it's not full of chemistry or 'jargon' so it isn't heavy going. Throughout, important points are reinforced in the margins and as 'post it' notes.

There has been a huge increase in the levels of childhood obesity in recent years. The media regularly reports on this problem, and it was this that led me to embark on the 'Healthy Eating and Lifestyle Promotion Tour of Wales' in 2000. This tour has become a regular event in my calendar and it was during one of the tours that it became clear to me that many parents had questions about their children's nutritional needs to which they wanted straightforward answers.

During my tours I met thousands of parents who obviously cared passionately about the health of their children, but were confused and overwhelmed by the conflicting dietary advice being presented in the media. There were also large numbers of parents who were not aware of the average daily energy requirements of children; I have therefore given this detail in Appendix 1 at the back of this book. Please do not get bogged down with the figures. Instead, have a little fun, do a little experiment using the figures as a reference. For one or two days, make a note of the calorie content of the processed foods you give your child/children (you will be able to find this information on food packaging). At the end of the day, total up the calories and compare the result with

. . . this book is written for you, in the hope that myths surrounding the issues of nutrition will be dispelled.

the information in Appendix 1. I did this experiment and was surprised at what I found; perhaps you too will be surprised at how many calories some processed foods contain. This short experiment may well make you more aware of or even re-enforce your awareness of just how many calories processed foods contain.

So this book is written for you, in the hope that myths surrounding the issues of nutrition will be dispelled. You will soon find that throughout the book I have repeated many points that I feel to be important. This is quite deliberate and is intended only to reinforce important information.

I have included a section (Chapter 12) devoted to the many questions posed to me during my tours. As you will see, the questions are many and varied and a large number of them refer to basic principles of nutrition. These are the very issues that become clouded by inappropriate advertising of foods that do not contribute to health and the conflicting and confusing information that we, as consumers, are bombarded with almost daily.

We as parents should be able to recognise the myths surrounding nutrition. Simply remember that children who are fed a diet of good wholesome foods and who are active are less likely to become overweight and suffer from a range of illnesses later in life.

Chapter 1

Setting the scene

My reason for writing this book is to target obesity in children, but it is not simply about weight loss (fat loss) for the sake of being thinner; it's about fat loss in the promotion of health. So health promotion in children is the aim of the book.

Millions of people are on diets, and they are spending billions of pounds on self-help, quick-fix books, diet drinks and foods, almost anything relating to weight-loss.

It's no wonder that the weight-loss industry is a booming one. Many, if not all, diets could be considered fad diets since most do not work in the long term because they are not sustainable. The promises of easy weight-loss diets are false and will not result in long-term success. Of course, many will result in weight loss early in the diet and give false hope because most of this weight loss is not fat loss but water loss.

As a loving parent I do not believe in dieting, and I would advise all parents, never to put children on a diet without the say so from a doctor or paediatric dietician (i.e. unless there are medical reasons for doing so). Dieting does not work in the long term because it results in a yo-yo effect where weight is lost then gained then lost then re-gained and so on. This is because as we reduce food to lose weight, our bodies recognise the drop in energy (calories) and so slow down the rate at which the calories consumed are burned off as energy. In this way our body is protecting itself in order to survive for longer. In other words our metabolic rate is reduced, and a low metabolic rate means we may find it harder to control weight gain. In this situation our body becomes more efficient at storing energy, i.e. as soon as more food is eaten it is more easily stored as fat and we put on weight. So, simply reducing calories is no guarantee that weight loss will take place.

Dieting often results in a yo-yo effect

We need to stimulate our metabolic rate which will burn off the calories we consume. Think of it as tricking our bodies not to go into this 'survival mode'. There are a number of things we can do to ensure this, and basically eating foods that require more energy to be broken down (i.e. unrefined foods) together with increasing physical activity are what it's all about. As parents who care about the health and well being of our children, we should lead by example, not only in the foods that we eat but also by the things that we do. For example, I always snacked on fruit in front of my daughter and while doing so encouraged her to do the same. When she was younger, my wife and I involved her in the washing of fruit and sometimes even cutting it into smaller pieces, e.g. for a fruit salad. We found that by getting our daughter involved she became less resistant to trying a whole variety of fruits.

Good nutrition coupled with suitable physical activity is essential for good health

. . . by getting our daughter involved in preparing food she became less resistant to trying a whole variety of foods.

Childhood obesity appears to increase with each generation, mainly as a result of poor nutrition and lack of physical activity. It's actually thought that if these increases are not dealt with then we will be in a position where obese children in the school playground will outnumber healthy weight children. This will only continue until the obese children eventually succumb to the diseases associated with obesity including heart disease and diabetes. It is wise to remember that even slim children are at risk of these problems unless they are introduced to good nutrition complemented by appropriate physical activity. As parents and carers, we play an essential role in establishing these lifestyle and dietary changes.

With respect to nutrition we are often very confused and it's hardly surprising because we are bombarded daily, via media articles and reports, with advice on a multitude of aspects relating to diet and nutrition. These are at best confusing, often conflicting, and not always based on good quality evidence. At worst they can be based on a frank misinterpretation or misunderstanding of nutrition science. This constant diet-a-day barrage creates a ping-pong effect of contradictory dietary advice which can leave us as parents with more questions than answers.

One of the consequences of this contradictory advice is that we may well end up believing that the 'experts' keep changing their minds. We therefore would probably continue with our unhealthy eating habits. There is also a worrying trend whereby individuals with no formal training or qualifications offer nutrition and dietary advice. Often, this advice is linked to the sale of supplements or specific foods. The media frequently use sports personalities, pop stars or film stars to promote a food not associated with health, e.g. crisps. Children are easily influenced by such promotions and we as parents need to be aware of this.

Dieting in its everyday sense will be shown not to be as important in promoting health as it is in losing weight. This is not to say that weight control is not important because weight control is very important with respect to health. The problem is with the use of the word 'diet', which implies food restriction. Food restriction is not a good idea as often it results in cravings which can make weight control difficult.

We need to realise that our children should not be put on food restriction diets in an attempt to get them to shed weight, because that may deprive them of valuable nutrients. Instead, good nutrition with regular physical activity will promote the building of muscle tissue. It's worth noting here that body fat does not require energy but muscle does. Encouraging our children to use their muscles by playing or running around, will help them use the energy supplied by their food, and therefore will promote health and improve weight control.

Cravings are the enemy when trying to control weight, and I don't know of any dieter who has not experienced overwhelming cravings and it is often the sugary, fatty foods they crave.

Basically, the foods our children eat are converted to glucose which is then used to produce energy. We can think of this in the same way as petrol fuels a car. What happens when you keep adding petrol to your car without using it? The tank (where the petrol is stored) over-flows. Our bodies are obviously different. Any glucose not used for energy will be stored (as glycogen) to be used later. When we do not need more glycogen, i.e. when the stores are full, additional food consumed is then converted to fat.

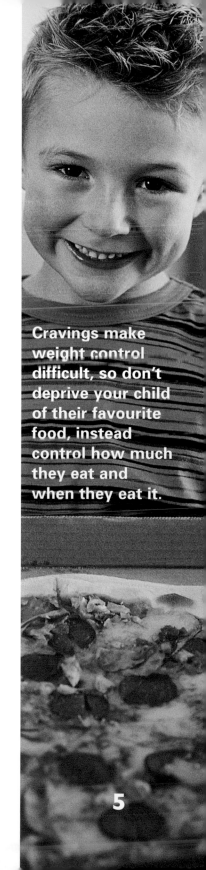

Cravings make weight control difficult, so don't deprive your child of their favourite food, instead control how much they eat and when they eat it.

5

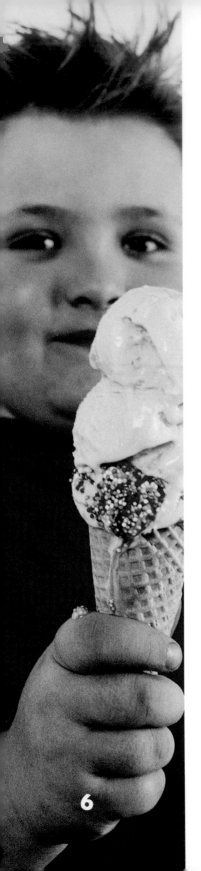

It's physical activity (similar to running the car engine) that helps prevent the build up of excess fat stores by stimulating the breakdown of the glycogen to glucose. The glucose is taken to our muscles and used by our muscles to fuel the activity.

We get an increase in blood glucose following consumption of food, especially if the food is high in sugar or is heavily processed. It's the increase in blood glucose levels which triggers our bodies to produce insulin. This release of insulin into the blood controls blood glucose levels, and also is what gives us our cravings for more sugary foods to take our blood sugar back up again. If these cravings are indulged, the excess sugar is likely to end up as stored fat; in other words we become overweight or obese.

Eating sugary foods results in cravings for more sugary foods

Chapter 2

Diet and health – the basic building blocks

Contrary to the impression we may have gained from the media, nutrition is not very complicated and there is certainly no voodoo-like magic to the way it works. The foods we consume are made up of carbohydrates, proteins and fats. These are called the macronutrients, which are the nutrients we need in large amounts. In addition, vitamins and minerals are required and these are essential if we are to be healthy. Vitamins and minerals are called micronutrients and they are required in small amounts only. Water is essential to all living things, and this is found in most groups and makes up a large proportion of our bodies.

In terms of energy consumption, proteins should make up around 15–20% of our diet, carbohydrates around 50–55% and fats around 30% (see Figure 2.1). Of the fat, no more than 10% should be saturated fat, which are usually animal fats like butter and lard. Vitamins and minerals are found within all these groups and a balanced diet should deliver all in adequate amounts.

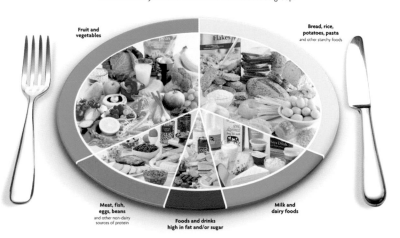

The eatwell plate

FOOD STANDARDS AGENCY
food.gov.uk

Use the eatwell plate to help you get the balance right. It shows how much of what you eat should come from each food group.

Fruit and vegetables

Bread, rice, potatoes, pasta
and other starchy foods

Meat, fish, eggs, beans
and other non-dairy
sources of protein

Foods and drinks
high in fat and/or sugar

Milk and dairy foods

Figure 2.1

Nutrition plate – the foods shown in the largest slices on the plate are the foods we should consume often, the foods shown on the smallest slice should be limited in our diets.

A healthy diet has to fulfil two objectives:

1. It must provide sufficient energy and nutrients to maintain normal body functions, and permit growth and replacement of body tissues.

2. It must offer protection against risk of disease and promote optimum body weight.

A supply of energy is a basic need of our bodies; without it we would die in weeks. This energy comes from carbohydrate, fat and protein. Because the need for energy is high, if sufficient energy is not obtained from the diet the body will start to break down its own reserves in order to meet its energy needs. Initially it will make use of fat stores, but as the energy deficit increases muscle will be broken down and used as a fuel supply. Muscle breakdown must be avoided and this is another reason to avoid starvation-type diets.

Carbohydrate

Dietary carbohydrate (sugars and starches) is broken down to glucose in the body (digestion) and is the most readily available source of energy to the body. Carbohydrates are our body's primary source of energy and mainly come from plant foods such as cereals, grains, fruits, vegetables, and legumes (peas and beans). Carbohydrates can be 'slow acting' or 'fast acting'.

The fast acting carbohydrates, sometimes referred to as simple carbo-hydrates, are sweeter in taste and commonly found in highly processed foods – these are not good foods. Examples of foods high in fast acting carbohydrates include cakes, biscuits and sweets. Foods rich in fast acting carbohydrates are prized for their sweetness but are not that nutritious, they are completely and rapidly digested and are a cause of dental caries. Consumption of these foods is also responsible for food (sugar) cravings.

Slow acting carbohydrates, sometimes referred to as complex carbohydrates, are less refined or processed and are much better for our children (and us!). Examples of slow acting carbohydrate-rich foods include many unprocessed foods such as legumes (beans and lentils), vegetables, unprocessed wholegrain cereals and seeds. These are nutritious foods which contain vitamins, minerals and fibre.

Fruit and vegetables are a great source of vitamins and fibre.

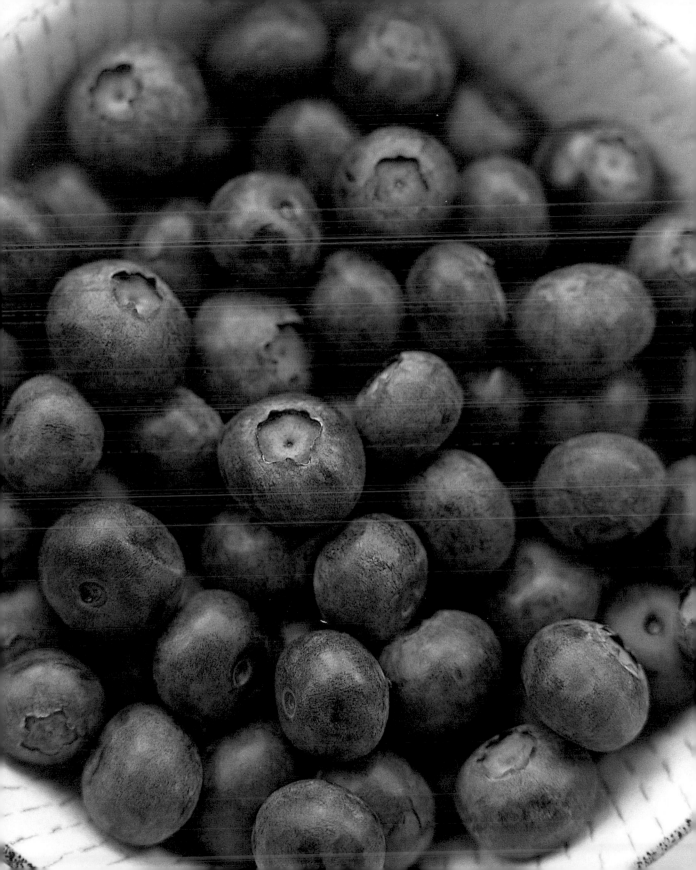

When we consume carbohydrates, our bodies break them down into glucose. This glucose ends up in our blood stream and is diverted to those parts of our bodies which require it for energy, e.g. our muscles and our brains. The hormone insulin effectively takes the glucose out of our blood to the muscles, and in this way controls our blood sugar levels. The digestion and absorption of slow release carbohydrate-rich foods (i.e. starches) are slower than the fast release carbohydrate foods (i.e. sugars), producing a much slower and more sustained blood glucose and insulin response. These foods are therefore considered to contribute to health more than the simple or fast acting carbohydrate-rich foods.

Slow release carbohydrates are much better for our children than simple carbohydrates

Many of you will have heard of the glycaemic index (GI) of foods in the media. High-GI carbohydrates are those which when consumed result in a rapid increase in blood glucose followed by a large release of insulin. High-GI foods are typically refined or processed foods where the skins or fibres have been removed and it's the removal of this fibre that allows our bodies to release the sugars from the food more quickly.

There is more information relating to the GI of foods later in this book.

Combining foods, e.g. high-GI foods with low-GI foods will slow down the overall sugar release, and this can be very useful when we plan our children's meals. As a general rule, foods with a high-GI do not promote health. On the other hand, low-GI carbohydrates result in the need for a slower release of insulin due to the slower release of glucose into the blood. Examples of low- and high-GI foods are given in Appendix 3 at the back of this book, but the table opposite defines the differences between low-GI, medium-GI and high-GI foods. Low GI foods are associated with reduced blood glucose, insulin and fat levels.

Dietary sources of carbohydrates

Excellent sources of carbohydrate include fruit, vegetables, whole grain products and many products based on oats, e.g. porridge. These foods are excellent food choices and we should encourage our children to consume them often (a minimum of five portions of fruit and vegetables

High glycaemic index foods	Moderate glycaemic index foods	Low glycaemic index foods
GI >70	GI 56–69	GI < 55
potatoes	wholemeal bread	milk
glucose	soft drinks	unripe banana
carrots	brown rice	apples
raisins	popcorn	fructose
croissants	bananas	flavoured yoghurt
shredded wheat	Special K cereal	beans
rice crispies	pastry	plums
cornflakes	sucrose	peanuts
	All-Bran cereal	fresh peaches
	low fat ice cream	
	kiwi fruit	

Table 2.1

Some examples of high, moderate and low GI foods

daily, e.g. two of fruit and three of vegetables). Highly processed and refined foods, e.g. cakes, biscuits and sweets, are poor sources and need to be restricted in our children's diets. When my daughter was young, I found it very useful not to have these highly processed foods in the house so that temptation was not a problem: 'out of sight out of mind'. Instead there was always a plentiful supply of fruit and yoghurts for snacking.

Fat

Dietary fat is a concentrated form of energy and also provides essential fatty acids necessary for the construction of cell membranes and many other functions. Fat is perceived to be a bad word; it conjures up all sorts of negatives in relation to health, and engenders an enormous amount of confusion and contradiction. Fat is an essential part of our diets. In addition to fat being used as a source of energy, it protects us from the cold, acts as a shock absorber for our organs and keeps our skin healthy.

It may also surprise you that consuming fat does not necessarily make you fat. It's the type and quantity of fat consumed that is the real issue. The type of fat consumed makes no difference to the energy density (all fats carry 9 kcal per gram) but the type of fat consumed has a significant effect on health, especially heart health.

Whether a fat is saturated or unsaturated is one way we differentiate between fats. Fats which are animal in origin are in general more saturated than vegetable fats and are therefore harder at room temperature.

As a general rule, restrict saturated fats in the diet, these are associated with high cholesterol and heart disease.

Carbohydrates =
3.75–4 kcal per gram

Protein =
4 kcal per gram

Fat =
9 kcal per gram

Unsaturated fats

Unsaturated fats are likely to be oils, and are healthier than saturated fats. This is especially true of the unsaturated fats found in oily fish and vegetable oils like olive oil. Unsaturated fats of the types found in oily fish (called omega 3s) are good for the heart because they reduce the bad cholesterol and increase the good cholesterol. Most vegetable oils are unsaturated, and such fats come in two types, they are monounsaturated and polyunsaturated.

Not all fats are bad . . .

Monounsaturated fats are good fats; they reduce bad cholesterol (LDL-Cholesterol) which is linked to coronary heart disease. This is evidenced by the Mediterranean diet, which relies on olive oil, nuts and other fatty foods, which typically are of the unsaturated type. Good sources of unsaturated fats include olive and rapeseed oils, walnuts and almonds.

. . . not all carbohydrates are good

There are two kinds of polyunsaturated fats. They are the omega-6 fats and the omega-3 fats. Omega-6 fats are found in vegetable oils such as corn, soy-bean and safflower oils. Our children are likely to be getting quite a lot of omega-6 fats in their diet because the food industry uses a lot of soy-bean oil. Omega-6 fats do lower cholesterol a little, but they lower both the bad (LDL) and the good (HDL) cholesterol.

Omega-3 fats have a much more powerful effect when it comes to lowering the bad cholesterol, and they do not lower the good cholesterol which is good news. Omega-3 fats therefore have a much more beneficial effect when it comes to protecting the heart against disease. Our bodies are not able to make these omega-3 fats, so we must get them from the foods we consume. The best source is from oily fish like mackerel, salmon, herring and sardines. We as parents should encourage our children to consume oily fish at least twice a week.

As a rule if a fat is hard at room temperature it is less good for our health.

Saturated fats

These are the bad fats, and high levels of consumption will raise the bad cholesterol more than anything else in our diet. Saturated fats are typically hard at room temperature, unlike the unsaturated fats which are typically oils at room temperature. The most common saturated fats include butter, lard and the fat that surrounds red meat. You will have noticed that all three are from animals and animals are the main suppliers of saturated fats. However, there are always exceptions and saturated fats can be found from vegetable sources, examples include cocoa butter (therefore it's found in chocolate) and palm oil which is often used in the manufacture of biscuits and other baked goods. These are every bit as bad for us as the saturated fats from animal sources. We should try to keep to a minimum the amount of saturated fats we feed our children.

Saturated fats are used in food products because they offer a longer shelf-life than when unsaturated fats are used. When we, the public, got wise to their use and started to prefer products made using unsaturated fats and rejecting the ones made using saturated fats, the food industry had to respond. What they did was to find a way of using the more acceptable oils and they did this by using a process called hydrogenation.

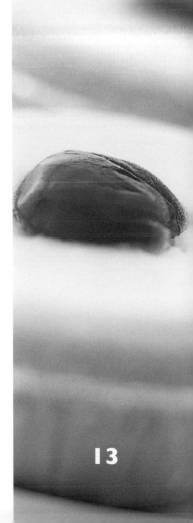

Hydrogenated fats are found in many baked products such as cakes and biscuits, these fats are bad for our hearts.

13

This process converts oils to fats by adding hydrogen to the unsaturated fats and using high temperatures to do so.

Hydrogenated fats are very unhealthy, so look out for them on food labels.

Hydrogenated fats are very good at prolonging the shelf life of products that contain them, but are the worst type of fats we could possibly consume because the process of hydrogenation results in the production of what are called trans-fats. Trans- fats are particularly bad for our hearts. They lower levels of good cholesterol and at the same time raise the levels of bad cholesterol in our blood. Trans-fats are not always listed on food labels so it's not always easy to tell which foods contain them. However, (and here's a good tip) we should read the labels on packaged foods and look for 'hydrogenated' or 'partially hydrogenated' fats in the ingredient list. If we see these, we can safely assume that the food will contain trans-fats, which should be avoided. Typically, a lot of baked products, including biscuits and cakes, will be made from hydrogenated fats. In fairness to the biscuit industry, they are looking to use alternative fats so look for them on the shelves.

The majority of fat in most western diets is in the form of 'invisible fats', i.e. fats incorporated into food products such as biscuits, cakes and most convenience or fast foods. This is one reason why these foods need to be restricted in our children's diet. It's so easy to give our children foods with these hidden fats, so it is worth while taking some time to read food labels. I consider it essential to get to grips with what's in our children's foods so I have included more information on reading food labels later in the book. If you would like to read more on food labels then go to Chapter 10.

Compared with carbohydrate or protein, fats are digested, absorbed and transported in our bodies differently because they do not mix well with water. Most people think of dietary fat as something to be avoided, however, some dietary fat is very important for good health. Fats help keep the skin and other tissues soft and pliable. The body uses fat to store as extra energy, which can be used to provide fuel to the working muscles. Fat stored as adipose tissue pads the body and protects the organs, and adipose tissue is an efficient way to store extra energy in a small space.

. . . **It is worth while taking some time to read food labels.**

Dietary sources of fat

Nuts (not suitable for young children because of the risk of choking and nut allergies), seeds and other vegetable sources, some margarines (take care with those containing hydrogenated fats) and fish are good sources of dietary fats. It's worth considering that nuts are so energy dense that spreads made from them, e.g. nut-butter, are a great deal more nutritious than margarines. After all, margarines are processed foods. Poor sources include those foods which contain hidden fats such as cakes, biscuits, pies, pasties and processed meats. As a general rule of thumb, vegetable fats are better for us than animal fats.

Protein

Protein provides amino acids which are essential for growth and continuous replacement of body tissues. There has been a great deal of confusing information regarding intakes of dietary protein, e.g. some people do not believe that consuming excess protein is a factor in weight control. Even though protein needs more energy to convert it to fat in the body it does contain calories (4 kcals per gram – similar to carbohydrate) so therefore can contribute to weight gain. The quantity of protein we and our children, consume does not have a significant effect on cholesterol levels but the source of the protein does. Meat and dairy products are good sources but they can also be good sources of saturated fats, which are thought to increase levels of cholesterol in the blood.

That said, proteins are an essential part of our diets and they play a very important role in repair and building of body tissue, e.g. muscle. Protein-rich foods are very good at making us feel fuller so we should encourage our children to eat some protein at every meal. Many foods that are mostly carbohydrate, e.g. bread and cereals, do contain low quality (low biological value) protein. Inadequate protein intake is most likely to occur in those

Protein supplements are not required if a balanced diet is consumed

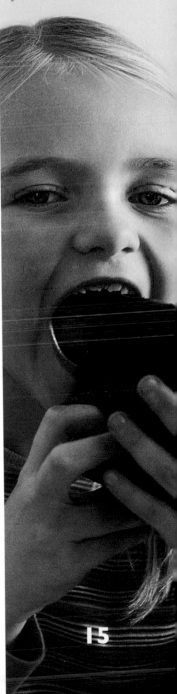

Poor sources include those foods which contain hidden fats such as cakes, biscuits, pies, pasties and processed meats.

15

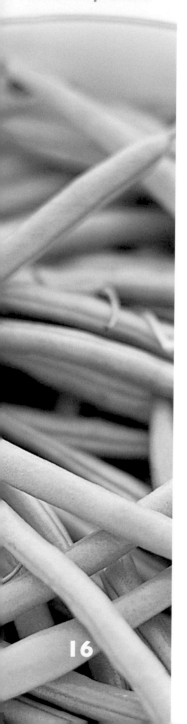

Legumes (peas and beans) are a good source of protein.

individuals who have particular pre-existing conditions, for example:

● where there is a need for an increase in protein, e.g. during periods of rapid growth in childhood

● where total energy intake is inadequate, e.g. among dieters

● where the diet includes only a narrow range of foods, e.g. in adolescents and vegetarians.

A balanced diet, i.e. a diet including foods from a wide variety of sources (fruit, vegetables, nuts, whole grain products and seeds) will provide an adequate intake of protein.

Dietary sources of protein

While meat (especially chicken and turkey), fish and dairy products contain high levels of protein, other good sources include cereals, grains, nuts and legumes. In addition, small amounts of protein can be found in some fruits, e.g. apricots, blueberries, and apples, and some vegetables, e.g. asparagus and green beans. Lacto-ovo-vegetarians (people who eat eggs and dairy products) can get their protein from foods like beans, nuts, soy products, eggs and dairy products, while vegans (people who do not eat animal products of any kind) can get their protein from beans, nuts, soy products and other plant sources of protein.

Vitamins, minerals and trace elements

These are required by the body in order for it to function efficiently. Most are only required in very small or even trace amounts. They do not provide energy so they cannot sustain life alone. However, without vitamins, minerals and trace elements, body functions will be impaired, body systems will malfunction, disease may result and life will be threatened. You can find more information on vitamins and minerals later in the book; see Chapters 7 and 8.

Dietary fibre

Fibre refers to the unabsorbed residues of plant food. The value of fibre lies in the fact that it is not absorbed/digested by the body. Dietary fibre helps to maintain normal bowel function and increases the feeling of being full, so consumption of adequate amounts is an important consideration when planning meals. There are two types of fibre, soluble and insoluble. It's the insoluble fibre (with extra drinking water) that will help prevent our children getting constipated, and the soluble fibre will help control cholesterol levels in the blood. A diet high in fruit, vegetables, seeds, wholegrain products and oats will ensure our children consume sufficient fibre. It's worth pointing out here that for dietary fibre to be really effective our children need to drink plenty of water.

For dietary fibre to be really effective our children need to drink plenty of water.

Salt

Our children should be encouraged not to add salt to their food as its present consumption is thought to be too high. Excess salt contributes to high blood pressure (hypertension), and heart disease. Reducing the addition of salt to foods during cooking is also recommended, and it's a good idea to take the salt cellar off the table to remove the temptation of adding extra salt. Take care with processed foods as these are notoriously high in salt.

Fluid (water)

Water is a vital component of a healthy diet; without it survival time is limited to a few days. Chronic dehydration can result in a number of ill-effects, such as constipation, increased risk of renal stone formation and mental confusion. Acute dehydration (e.g. due to severe vomiting or diarrhoea) is life-threatening. Children should be encouraged to drink plenty of water (6–8 glasses) daily and this should be spread throughout the day.

Processed foods can be very high in salt

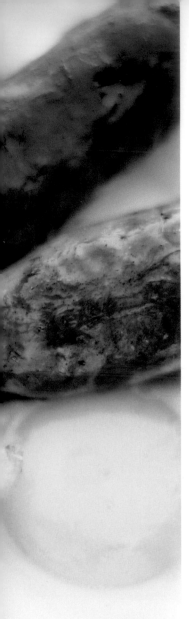

Something about cholesterol

While cholesterol is not considered a food, it's very important as high levels of cholesterol in the blood are thought to contribute to heart disease. Even though cholesterol is thought of as the villain, you might be surprised to learn that in fact it is needed by the body and performs a number of functions, including the manufacture of important hormones such as oestrogen and testosterone, and as an important component of cell structure.

Consuming a diet high in saturated fat is likely to increase cholesterol levels and therefore chances of heart disease.

We get problems when the amount of cholesterol in our blood rises to a high level, when it can cause blocked arteries and contribute to heart disease. Cholesterol gets into our bodies via two sources. Firstly, our bodies make it and, secondly, we can consume it in our foods (called dietary cholesterol). The main sources of dietary cholesterol are animal products and include eggs, meat, offal such as brains, kidney, whole milk, cheese and ice-cream.

We make all the cholesterol our bodies need, so the chances are if our diets contain high levels of cholesterol we will increase blood levels to an unhealthy level. While this is basically true, individuals react differently to dietary cholesterol based on the kinds of fat they consume (saturated or unsaturated) and their inherited responsiveness (genetics). It is, however, a good idea to prevent our children consuming high levels of cholesterol-rich foods.

The main sources of dietary cholesterol are animal products.

Chapter 3

Requirements of pre-school children

At home and prior to school age, our children's experiences of food are going to be limited by the family, and as a rule our eating habits will be the eating habits copied by our children. However, when our children start school they are exposed to different eating experiences. For example there may be breakfast clubs, school meals, sharing their packed lunches with friends and they may have access to tuck shops. Being exposed to these experiences will impact on their eating behaviour.

At different stages in our children's development there will be different rates of growth, e.g. during infancy, between the ages of six and eight years (often called the mid growth spurt), and at adolescence. Though the most significant changes take place during the adolescent stage, good nutrition is important at all stages of development. To ensure steady growth, energy requirements (from food) are higher in pre-pubertal children than they are in adults. Often the temptation is to offer high energy foods, e.g. biscuits or cakes, as snacking foods to 'keep them going' and in this way children develop poor eating habits which may be long lasting.

Young children have high energy and nutrient requirements relative to their size. Depending on growth rate and level of physical activity, they have an appetite which is variable and in addition they have a small stomach which prevents the consumption of large quantities of food at any one time. It is far better to encourage the consumption of several smaller meals with suitable snacks rather than giving fewer larger meals.

In order to meet the micronutrient (i.e. vitamins and minerals) requirements as well as energy requirements, much of the food should be of high nutrient density. High nutrient density means that the food is high in vitamins and minerals and not just high in for example sugar or

Good nutrition is very important at all stages of our children's development.

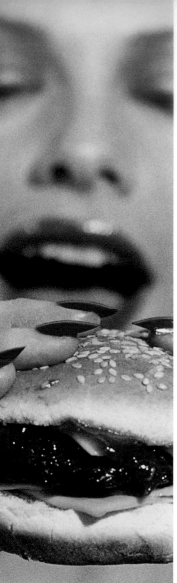

If we have bad eating habits, our children are likely to adopt similar habits.

fat. Fruit and vegetables are high in nutrients whereas a packet of sweets is not.

Nutrient dense foods are high in vitamins and minerals, whereas energy dense foods are high in calories.

Ideally, our children should eat most meals at the table with the rest of the family and family discussions should be encouraged. Eating meals whilst watching television should be discouraged, such habits may lead to over-eating and poor social skills. Good eating habits will promote good communication skills, so family meal times are important. Our children should be encouraged to help with meal planning; for example, we could involve them in food shopping. They can help in meal preparation by washing fruit etc. This will not only develop their social skills, but will also demonstrate the importance of food and the contribution a healthy diet makes to health and well being. A summary of nutritional tips is given in Appendix 4 at the back of this book.

Pre-school children are generally well nourished; they are taller and heavier than those of 25 years ago when children consumed around 17% more energy than today's children of the same age. Never the less today's children are bigger (fatter) and the differences are related to the differences in the levels of physical activity. Today's children are less active!

It is very important that by the age of five years our children should be physically active at a level of at least moderate intensity for an hour every day. Physical activity does not mean formal exercise, activities such as skipping or kicking a ball around the garden are all important. At this age activities like watching a lot of television and playing computer games should be discouraged.

It's very important to encourage our children to be active, if possible for one hour a day, every day

Regard food high in sugar as treats which should not be consumed as a major part of our children's diet.

Carbohydrates

Though most pre-school children consume adequate energy for their needs, much of it tends to come from high-sugar and high-fat foods like biscuits, confectionery and sweets. These foods are low in micronutrients (e.g. vitamins) relative to their energy content, they do not contribute to positive health and they promote dental caries (tooth decay). These foods should be limited and they should not form an important part of our children's diets.

In addition, sweet foods result in cravings, which make weight control difficult and result in rapid and high insulin production which has long-term implications for health. As I have already said, the best foods to deliver the best carbohydrates are the unrefined or unprocessed foods like whole grain products (e.g. brown bread, brown rice and rolled oats). These foods contain slow release carbohydrates which take longer for the digestive system to break down and this means that sugars will be released to the bloodstream more slowly, reducing sugar cravings. Most children tend to like sweet foods and there are a number of possible reasons for this. They may have been offered sweets at a very young age as a reward for being well behaved. A consequence of this is that they develop a liking for sweet sugary foods. Giving sweets as a reward is not a good idea, because it adds to the positive image of such foods. Offering sweets as an 'occasional' treat is more acceptable. Occasional could mean no more than once a week, perhaps at the weekend. A better reward for well-behaved children would be to give them a cuddle and let them know how important they are.

Fat

In young children, a diet including insufficient fat may result in insufficient energy. However, in order to reduce the risks of illnesses such as heart problems in later life, our children should be encouraged to progress towards a diet lower in fat-rich food. This means reducing foods like biscuits and cakes, the very foods young children tend to enjoy most. Semi-skimmed milk should not be introduced before the age of five years as it's too low in energy and vitamins. By the age of five years, dietary fat should make up no more than 35% of energy intake.

Do not offer sweets as a reward for good behaviour.

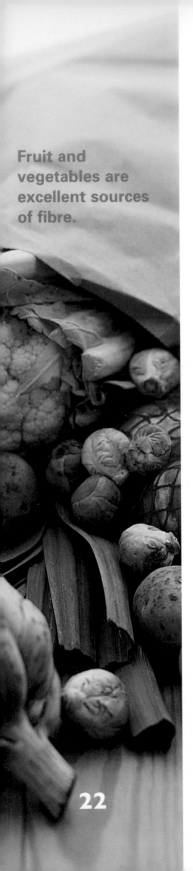

Fruit and vegetables are excellent sources of fibre.

Protein

We as parents should be aware that our children should eat protein at every meal if possible. This will help prevent over-eating. The recommended levels of protein for children are given in Appendix 8 at the back of this book. Dairy products are a good source, but if your child is sensitive to dairy products or has an allergy to the sugar lactose found in dairy products, then chicken, fish, red meat and seeds are excellent sources.

Fibre

There is no official recommendation for dietary fibre in young children, but they should have a lower intake than the 18g per day, which is recommended for adults. Pre-school children typically consume around 6g per day, which is a little low. Most of this fibre comes from potatoes and other vegetables. Fruit is not as big a part of children's diet as it should be, and our pre-school children should be encouraged to consume five small portions of fruit and vegetables daily as part of their normal diet. There is a relationship between fibre intake and regularity of bowel movements, and a healthy diet containing sufficient fibre should also contain sufficient water to enable the fibre to do its work through the digestive system, i.e. keep stools soft. Take care though: fibre is filling, so excessive consumption may result in insufficient energy intake.

Vitamins and minerals

Most children have adequate intakes of most vitamins, except vitamin A. For this vitamin, daily intakes are often below the recommended intake of 400 μg in many children. Milk and vegetables are the main sources of this vitamin, and young children tend not to consume large quantities of vegetables. It would be prudent in such cases for children of this age to be given a supplementary source of vitamin A, via Department of Health vitamin drops. In addition, the Department of Health recommends that children up to five years of age should be given supplements of vitamins A, C and D. I suggest you discuss this with your doctor or a paediatric dietician.

Many of the foods consumed by children in this age group are fortified with iron (e.g. breakfast cereals) and iron plus calcium (wheat flour). Cereal products are therefore a major source of these minerals. Another source of calcium is milk and milk products.

The contribution of milk and its products to calcium intake is highest in the youngest children and falls off as the child gets older. That said, milk is not thought to be a very good source of calcium because it does not have enough magnesium to balance it and help build healthy bones and teeth. The ideal calcium:magnesium ratio is 2:1, but the ratio in milk is 10:1. Nuts, seeds, dark green leafy vegetables, soy products and fish have a much better ratio. Calcium enriched cereal products are the other major source of calcium for children, and the proportion derived from this source increases with age. Later in this book you will find a summary of vitamins and minerals, their uses and recommended intakes. Remember though, the best way to take vitamins and minerals is in foods like fruit and vegetables, but bear in mind that the water soluble vitamins like vitamin C are easily destroyed by cooking so take care with cooking times and temperatures. It is often better to steam foods rather than boil them. In this way less of the vitamins are lost because steaming is a more efficient cooking method.

Don't over-cook foods as this will destroy vitamins

Healthy eating for pre-school children

Our children should be encouraged to try a variety of foods, and they will need to eat little and often. Appropriate snacks should be offered between meals to act as mini-meals. Children should be encouraged to sit at the table for all main meals. Take care with snacks – foods like crisps, chocolate bars and sugary drinks should be discouraged. Good choices of snack foods include fruit, raw carrot, breadsticks, wholewheat wholemeal currant buns or teacakes, breakfast cereals which are not sugar coated, yoghurt or fromage frais. The best drinks to serve between

Discourage sugar-coated cereals for our children's breakfast.

23

meals are milk or water, sugary drinks should be avoided. Food from all four main groups should be consumed daily, that is:

- bread, cereals and potatoes,
- fruit and vegetables,
- milk and dairy foods and
- meat and fish.

In the 5-a-day rule, potatoes do not count.

In order to provide the essential nutrients, especially calcium and iron, children like adults, should consume a minimum of five portions of fruit and vegetables per day (in the 5-a-day rule, potatoes do not count). Examples of suitable portions for a child under five years include 25ml of apple or orange juice diluted with water, a small banana or half an apple or pear, a small bowl of tinned fruit (own juice), 40g portions of broccoli, carrots, corn, green beans, peas or tomatoes. You will have noted that these portion sizes are smaller than the portion sizes for adults (80g). Foods containing peanuts should not be given to children below the age of three years, if a parent or sibling has a diagnosed allergy. Whole nuts should not be given to any child below the age of five years because of the risk of choking.

Common Dietary Problems in Pre-School Children

Fussy Eaters

At around the age of two years, food refusal often becomes an issue as the toddler begins to assert his or her independence. Young children should be encouraged to participate in self-feeding and to choose some food. If our children are allowed too much control however, nutritional problems are likely because too often they will choose high-sugar foods at the expense of fruit and vegetables. Usually, children will quickly pass through this phase of selective and faddy eating, but we as parents and carers will need to exert some tolerance as they do so.

During this phase, it may be advisable to give the child a multivitamin supplement designed for young children. This multivitamin should contain no more than the RNI (reference nutrient intake) for micronutrients (see Appendix 7). Remember though, discuss this with your doctor or a paediatric dietician. Take care with excessive consumption of sugary drinks, and grazing on high-sugar and high-fat foods should also be discouraged. Three meals with two or three snacks (with suitable snacking foods, e.g. fruit or yoghurt) should be the target. If our children dislike vegetables or other health promoting foods, it is sometimes helpful to continually offer those foods in small quantities as this often results in their eventual acceptance.

Dental Caries (Tooth Decay)

The widespread introduction of toothpaste containing fluoride is thought to have resulted in a significant reduction in the incidence of dental caries. However, take care because fluoride is a toxin and can cause dental fluorosis in large amounts. Young children from more deprived sectors of the population are more likely to be at risk from and have an increased prevalence of dental caries. Children should be encouraged to brush their teeth twice a day and this should be supervised.

Consumption of sugary foods and drinks should be reduced and kept to mealtimes only; they should never be consumed just prior to bedtime. Remember, at this age we are in control of our children's diet. If sugary, fatty or salty foods are not offered to our children then there is a very good chance that a taste for such foods will not develop.

Iron-Deficiency Anaemia

In socially disadvantaged groups and the immigrant population, iron-deficiency anaemia is common in pre-school children. Iron deficiency is associated with frequent infections, poor weight gain, delay in development and behavioural disorders. It is an important treatable condition in early childhood. It is usually of dietary origin, associated with late or inappropriate weaning and the early introduction of cow's milk. Cow's milk is not a good source of iron.

Fruit smoothies are an excellent way to get our children to consume fruits.

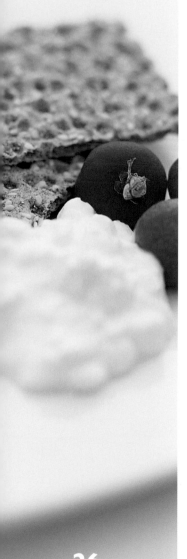

Snacking between meals with health promoting foods is important.

Foods like meat, fish, fruit and vegetables should be included daily. Liver is a good source of iron. Haem iron (found in meat) is much more readily absorbed than non-haem iron (found in vegetables). However, the absorption of iron from plant sources can be enhanced by the simultaneous consumption of vitamin C-rich foods and drinks, e.g. citrus fruit juices and tomatoes. Vitamin C increases iron absorption.

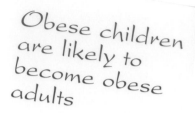

Obese children are likely to become obese adults

Obesity

Children of pre-school age are totally dependent on other people for their food therefore we as parents/carers can inadvertently encourage obesity in our children. Obesity is most often the result of over-consumption of high-energy foods, like biscuits, cakes, crisps, etc., coupled of course, with insufficient physical activity. There is a great temptation for us to insist that our young children eat everything on their plates; this is not a good idea. Such behaviour is effectively force feeding and teaches the child to overeat. It is far better to give smaller portions and if the child wants more let them ask.

Poor Appetite

In the absence of underlying disease, and if our children are growing normally, poor eating is unlikely to be a major problem. If our children appear healthy, management of the poor eater revolves around reassurance and education. Parents should be reminded that from birth to one year a child gains around 6kg (15lb), but during the following years the average weight gain is only 2kg (5lb) per year, in other words, the rapid growth and increases in food intake of a baby do not continue.

Many young children prefer drinking to eating and they readily fill themselves up with drinks. Therefore, we should avoid giving our children a drink one hour before a meal. This is not to suggest we reduce fluid intake throughout the day, but simply try to avoid our children drinking prior to a meal. Drinks should be offered at the end of a meal. If

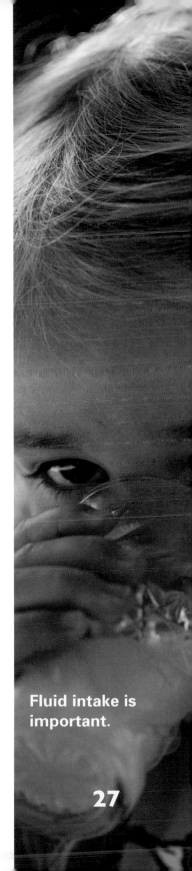

our children still drink from a bottle, a cup should be encouraged as this will decrease fluid intake. Small children need to snack between meals, so it's important that our children snack on appropriate foods, e.g. half a banana or plain biscuit. Crisps and chocolate biscuits are best avoided. We must never make our children finish a meal, and food not consumed should be removed without comment. Pre-school children's eating habits will often improve when they come into contact with other children, and once they start school they also tend to become more active, and this should be encouraged.

Diarrhoea

This is not uncommon, and the problem is thought to be due to immaturity of gut function and it often improves around the age of three to four years. Toddlers' diarrhoea is considered a harmless condition, and consumption of large quantities of fruit or fruit juice is a common cause, as the immature gut is inefficient at absorbing fructose (fruit sugar) resulting in what's termed osmotic diarrhoea. Excess sucrose (which is converted in the body to glucose and fructose) may have similar effects if consumed in large quantities. If our children consume a fibre-rich diet, then it would be prudent to reduce this, perhaps by reverting to refined foods for a short time, e.g. white bread etc. Remember always check with a doctor if your child develops diarrhoea.

Constipation

Constipation is defined as the infrequent passing of hard stools. Young children may become constipated, and in this case, consumption of high-fibre foods should be encouraged. It's important to choose foods which our children will enjoy, e.g. baked beans, whole grain breakfast cereals, or high fibre white bread. Unprocessed bran should not be given as it can cause bloating or flatulence and reduce the absorption of micronutrients, e.g. iron. Fluid intake is important, and poor drinkers should be encouraged to drink more water or diluted fruit juice. Physical activity will also help if your child is constipated. If the condition persists, you should check with your doctor.

Fluid intake is important.

27

Healthy eating recommendations for pre-school children

Dietary modifications to reduce fat intake and increase fibre intake are not recommended before the age of two years. At the age of five years however, the intake of energy from fat should not exceed 35% of total energy and possibly even less. Remember that pre-school-aged children must obtain sufficient energy and nutrients from the diet and this must not be compromised by a diet too low in fat or too high in fibre. The timing of the change from an infant high-fat, low-fibre diet to a diet which is lower in fat (where the fat has been replaced by slow acting carbohydrates, e.g. whole grain cereals) and also higher in fibre should be flexible. For children who gain weight slowly this change may not be appropriate until the age of five years.

We should encourage our children to eat fruit, vegetables and whole grain cereals daily e.g. rolled oats, flaked brown rice etc. A good guide is four portions of these foods daily at the age of two to three years, which should be increased to five daily portions at the age of five years. Remember, cereals should be of the whole grain type and the consumption of processed cereals should be minimised.

Milk or dairy products like yoghurt and fromage frais should be included each day and we should aim for two portions (cups) daily. Semi-skimmed milk (from five years onwards) and low fat dairy products should also be encouraged. Lean meats (take care with fatty meats) can be used in moderation, one to two portions daily, and oily fish like mackerel, herrings, sardines and tuna should be consumed at least once a week, better still twice. Non-meat and non-dairy protein foods should be encouraged. These will include peas, beans, baked beans and lentils.

Keep foods high in salt, fat and/or sugar and fried foods to a minimum

Remember, salty, sugary and fatty foods must be kept to a minimum. This does not mean they must never be consumed, but these foods should be thought of as treats and not as part of a health-

Lean meats can be used in moderation.

promoting diet. It is a good idea not to have these foods readily available in the house. In addition, remember to limit consumption of animal fats (saturated fats) and in particular foods containing hydrogenated or partially hydrogenated fats. Read food labels; these fats will be listed, but in any case they are commonly used in a large number of baked items like cakes and biscuits.

Do not give fried foods every day, in fact it is best to keep these foods to a minimum, e.g. no more than once per week (less if possible). When we do fry we should use the minimum amount of oil and never fry in hard margarine, butter, coconut oil or lard. Take care also with salt addition to food; we are all consuming far too much salt in our diets. Reduce levels during cooking and do not put salt on the table.

Encourage physical activity and discourage too much television, computer games etc. We need to find an activity our children enjoy; it does not have to be sport related though most children enjoy some forms of sport. Skipping, bike riding and swimming are all good activities.

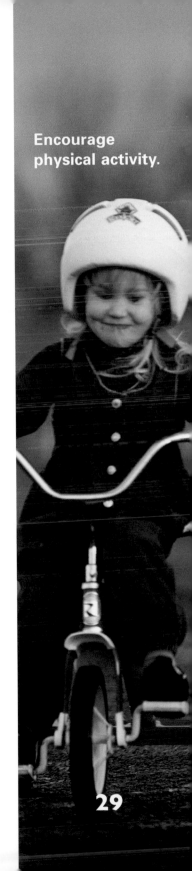

Encourage physical activity.

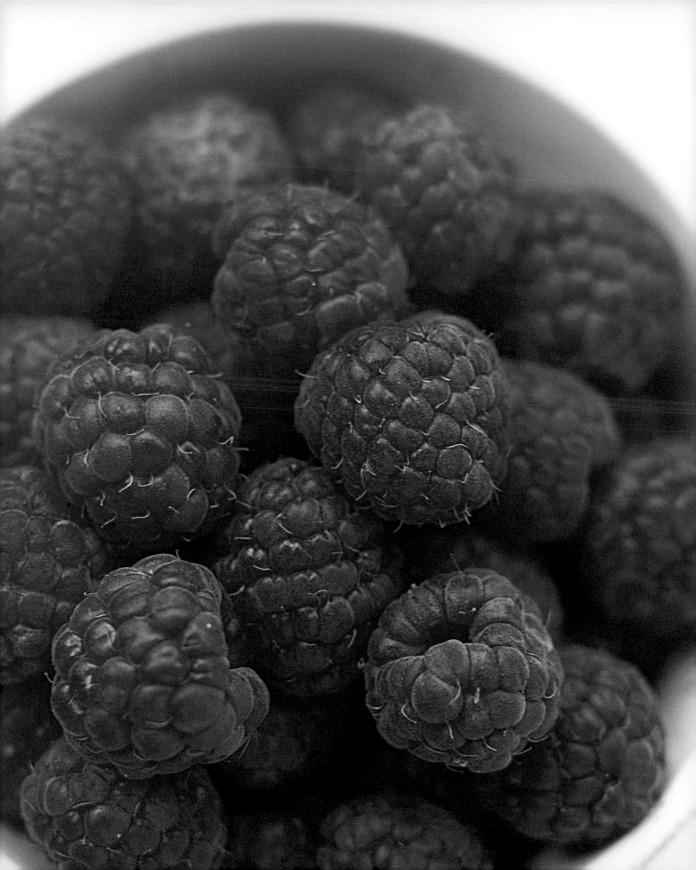

Chapter 4

Healthy eating for school-aged children

The eating habits of school-aged children are easily affected by outside influences, school dinners and visiting friend's homes. At this stage in their lives, we as parents lose some control over what our children eat, so we need to be aware of this.

Berries and other brightly coloured fruits are packed with goodness.

School-aged children should be encouraged to eat at least five portions of fruit and vegetables daily and also as wide a variety as possible and not simply the same fruits. We should try to get our children to eat brightly coloured fruit and vegetables, e.g. strawberries, raspberries and sprouts, these contain higher levels of the micronutrients that offer protection against illness and they also promote health. Nuts, seeds and wholegrain products are excellent sources of fibre and health-promoting fats and should be an important part of our children's diet.

We need to ensure that our children have breakfast every day, but we should stay away from sugar-coated cereals as these result in a sugar craving soon after they are eaten. Porridge is an excellent start to the day; try adding some chopped fruit in place of sugar. If our children will not eat a solid breakfast try a smoothie (see Appendix 5) which is very easily prepared and highly nutritious. My daughter has always insisted that she is unable to eat breakfast, so I introduced her to smoothies many years ago. She now drinks a very nutritious smoothie every morning and has often told me that she no longer has the lack of energy mid-day that she used to have.

During my tours of Wales, I actively promote home-made smoothies to both children and parents and these have always proved to be a hit with everyone. We should encourage our children to help in the making of

Berries and other brightly coloured fruits are packed with goodness.

If our children will not eat a solid breakfast try a smoothie.

them and this will increase the chance that they will consume them. I have found that even children who thought they did not like fruit were prepared to try them.

Snacking is also important to control blood sugar, but take care with the choice of food. Fruit, celery sticks, yoghurt and fromage frais are all excellent choices; crisps, cakes, biscuits and chocolate are poor choices.

When our children start school, we lose some control over what they consume. For instance, we have no control over school meals. Other factors may also be important – we may include a piece of fruit in our child's lunch box, but they may swap this for a bar of chocolate in the playground. In other words, there are a number of factors that may influence the eating behaviour of our children, and poor eating habits set early in life are likely to stay.

Common Dietary Problems in School-Aged Children

Compared to previous generations, today's children appear to have fewer health problems. That said, there is a concern that unhealthy lifestyles and diet are likely to lead to some serious problems in later life, such as heart problems, diabetes, high blood pressure and some cancers. Of significant importance with respect to these illnesses is obesity, so this will be discussed first.

Obesity

A large percentage of school-aged children are classed as either over-weight or obese, and this trend is increasing with each generation. Risks for childhood obesity have been reported to be excessive food intake, (often the wrong types of foods), high parental body weight, and of course lack of physical activity. As surprising as it might seem, young children may have concerns about their body weight, and some are on diets. The problem is worse for girls and we as parents should note that it is not a good idea to put our children on food-restricted diets without consulting a doctor. It is far more appropriate to offer good nutrition and

Obesity is a trend which is increasing with every generation

this means as wide a choice of wholesome unprocessed foods as possible, including plenty of fresh fruit and vegetables.

Young children are becoming more sensitive to body image, perhaps as a result of the images in magazines of thin models portrayed as those with the 'perfect' body. We need to be aware of this and not be tempted to put our children on a diet (unless advised to do so by a doctor). Thinness should not be the objective, but health should.

Under-weight

If our children are persistently very light, this needs to be investigated. Reasons for under-weight may include an underlying medical condition, poor appetite, family problems, concern about body image, and self-imposed dietary restriction. We should note if our children are not eating well, we need to be vigilant. Though eating disorders are not common in children they do occur and can be serious.

Dental Caries

Another common problem with young school children, particularly if fed a diet high in sugars, is dental caries. Care with food choices offered to our children can significantly reduce tooth decay. Consumption of sugary and acidic foods (e.g. some fizzy drinks) should be kept to a minimum.

Iron-Deficiency Anaemia

Although iron intake in pre-pubertal children is generally adequate, iron-deficiency anaemia does occur. Encouraging consumption of foods such as fortified breakfast cereals, dried fruits, red meat (take care with the fat) and baked beans will help. Iron uptake can be maximised by offering fruit juice with meals and avoiding foods which tend to hamper absorption, such as tea or high-fibre cereals.

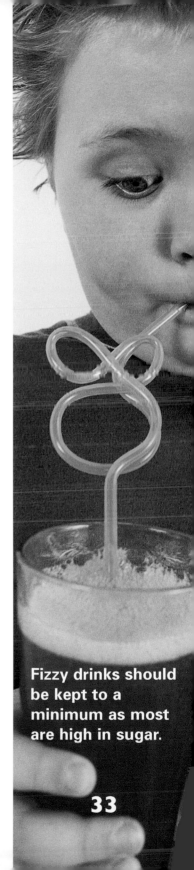

Fizzy drinks should be kept to a minimum as most are high in sugar.

33

Most children do not have food allergies but they may have a food intolerance.

Allergies and Intolerances

We often believe our children have 'allergies' or behavioural problems which are related to food. Most of these beliefs are likely to be unfounded, but our concerns need to be taken seriously by healthcare professionals to establish whether there is a basis for them. Food-exclusion measures should be undertaken under the supervision of a paediatric dietitian. Do not forget that removing foods which are major nutrient contributors, such as milk and dairy products, or wheat, can seriously compromise the nutritional status of young children.

Practical Advice

Three main meals and two to three snacks should be encouraged, but ensure snacking foods do not include high-sugar and high-fat foods typically liked by young school children. In addition, take care with salty foods. Currently it is widely accepted that we all consume far too much salt. Snacks should be based on unrefined starchy foods, e.g. wholemeal bread, fruit and fruit yoghurts. Examples of good snacking foods are given in Appendix 6 at the back of this book. Semi-skimmed milk should be encouraged and approximately half a litre of milk will meet the calcium requirements of the school-age child. We should never force our children to eat everything on their plate; this trains them to over-eat. Instead, we should offer smaller portions. Many parents believe it's in the best interest of the child to eat everything on their plate, but this is not true. This could have serious consequences as they get older, because over-eating results in excess weight gain and obesity. If we believe our children are not eating enough, e.g. they show signs of lethargy and lack of concentration, we need to see our doctors for advice.

Let's get our children interested in food, let them help with the shopping and meal preparation.

Our children should be involved in meal preparation; let's encourage them to help wash fruit and vegetables and get them to help lay the table etc. Children should know that mealtimes are important and ideally they should eat at the table with the rest of the family. Too many children

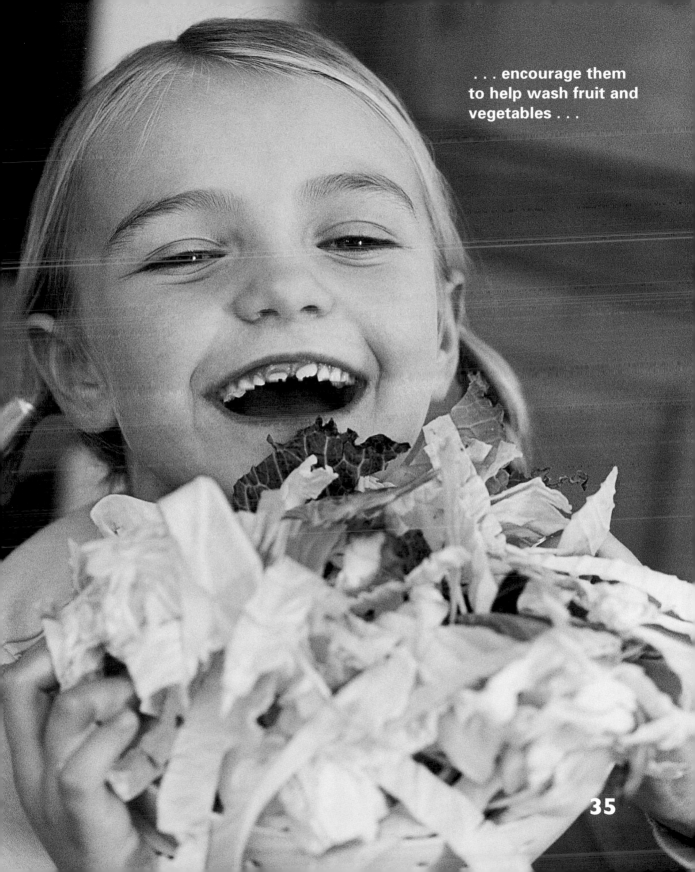

. . . encourage them to help wash fruit and vegetables . . .

35

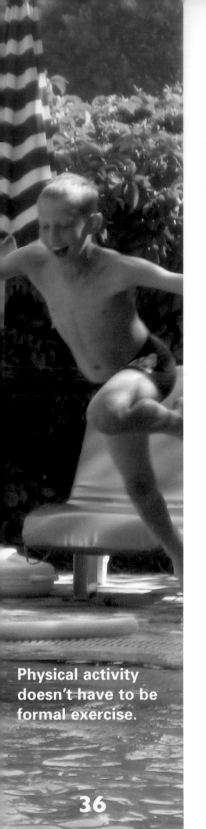

Physical activity doesn't have to be formal exercise.

eat their meals whilst watching television, this will often result in over-eating because children eat faster when watching television.

We should take our children shopping with us but avoid doing so when they are hungry because they will be tempted towards the chocolate and crisps.

When at the shop, take advantage of the opportunity to show them the varieties of fruit and vegetables available but stay away from the fast food aisles.

Physical activity should be encouraged, and this does not have to mean sport or formal exercise. Walking, swimming, playing and cycling are all good forms of physical activity. Children should be encouraged to take part in physical activity for approximately one hour a day. The activity should make them just out of breath, but they should still be able to hold a conversation. Regular bouts of physical activity can:

- increase levels of good cholesterol (HDL)
- lower high blood pressure
- help improve body composition by burning body fat
- promote healthy blood sugar levels
- boost the immune system
- improve mood.

Encourage our children to enjoy physical activity

Chapter 5

Healthy Eating for Adolescents

The principles that apply to school-aged children also apply to adolescents. At least five portions of fruit and vegetables should be consumed daily, taken from as large a variety as is possible. A portion for this age group is 80g. Remember that potatoes do not count and fruit juice only counts once. Unrefined and unprocessed foods should be main choices, with refined foods consumed only as treats and even then not often. Excellent choices of health-promoting foods include fruits, vegetables, fish (especially oily fish), nuts, oats and seeds (e.g. sunflower and pumpkin). With increasing pressure for teenagers to do well at school, there is often a great deal of homework which can often result in poor snacking habits during study time. It's crucial that this age group are aware of the problems associated with a poor diet and are encouraged to take responsibility for their health. Perhaps we pay too much attention to academia and not enough to long-term health?

Common Dietary Problems in Teenagers and Young Adults

Adolescents tend to be more influenced by peer pressure than by pressures from parents and school. In fact, messages about health from schools and other bodies of authority are often seen by adolescents as less important than the views of their peers. Intake of certain nutrients, for example riboflavin, vitamin D, calcium and iron, have been shown in several studies to be low in children aged around eleven to eighteen years, so take care with food choices, especially with girls. Puberty is a very important time for the deposition of calcium in bones and over half of adult peak bone mass (density) is accrued at this time. Low levels of calcium increase the risk of osteoporosis later in life.

Perhaps we pay too much attention to academia and not enough to long-term health.

37

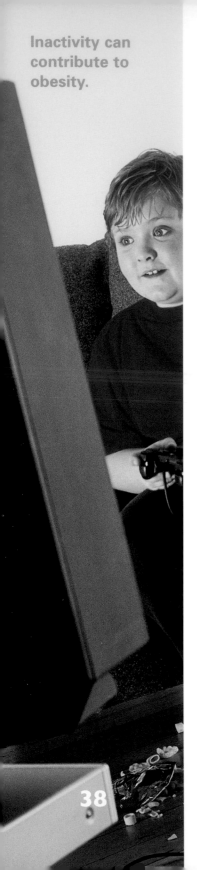

Inactivity can contribute to obesity.

Adolescents also tend to consume high levels of saturated fats, sugar and salt, resulting in the main from snacking on the wrong types of foods and consuming high levels of convenience foods coupled with low intakes of fruit and vegetables. In this age group, not only is obesity a problem but it is the age when eating disorders like anorexia also may become a problem.

Adolescence is a time when fat is deposited in girls as a natural process.

Obesity

As with younger children, teenagers who are inactive and/or consume a poor diet suffer obesity or over-weight. During adolescence, fat is deposited rapidly, so it should not surprise you that this is an important stage for the development of obesity. In boys, fat is commonly deposited around the mid section, while in girls it is commonly deposited in the breast and hip regions. Don't worry, this deposition of fat is natural and should not result in obesity. However, if our children are inactive and consume a poor diet, excess fat is likely to be deposited and there will be a greater risk of obesity.

In later life, excess fat has a major impact on quality and even duration of life. For the teenager, being over-weight may result in bullying and reduced social development. Let's not forget, that it's around this age that there may be a preference for television, computer games, etc., and if this is the case, then physical activity is likely to be significantly reduced.

Inappropriate Slimming

At this age body image becomes very important, so important in fact that we as parents need to take great care, if our children (particularly daughters) are dieting, that they do not go too far with weight loss. I have already said that dieting is not a good idea; it's far better to encourage healthy eating habits, which means more unprocessed foods, more fruit and vegetables and less sugary foods. Dieting in the strict sense of the word is often at the expense of health.

What our children consume should promote optimum health. Some of the slimming techniques that may be used are also cause for concern, with laxatives, diuretics and vomiting all being employed for quick results. Unsupervised and unnecessary slimming can result in low

Dieting may result in health problems

micronutrient (vitamins, minerals and trace elements) intake, as the diet often involves missing meals, particularly breakfast. Breakfast is an important meal, and should never be skipped. Parents and children should get up earlier if necessary to ensure there is plenty of time for breakfast. Teenagers enjoy smoothies as much as younger children and they provide an excellent breakfast for teenagers who refuse to eat a solid breakfast.

Eating Disorders

An excessive concern about body image is likely to end up being more serious. Adolescence is the peak age of onset of eating disorders such as anorexia nervosa and bulimia nervosa. We should note the signs of under-eating and consult a doctor if suspicions are raised. The best way to improve body image is to encourage more physical activity with consumption of health-promoting foods, e.g. fruit, vegetables and other unrefined foods.

Diet Experimentation

Adolescence is also a period of experimentation with diet. Many young people try special diets such as vegetarian or vegan and this in itself is not a problem. However, if the diets are poorly planned and imbalanced, the result can be an inadequate intake of some micronutrients. Common pitfalls are failure to consume foods which sufficiently compensate for the loss of iron from the diet, and, in the vegan diet, alternative sources of protein need to be found, e.g. soy products.

Body image, in particular thinness, is important to young teenagers.

Alcohol

Most adolescents will try alcohol at some time. High alcohol intake is a cause for concern for both health and social reasons, and young people have less ability to deal with alcohol consumption than fully mature adults and are more susceptible to its adverse effects. Regular alcohol consumption will displace more nutrient-dense foods from the diet, and easily lead to weight gain.

Alcohol comes second in the league table for energy (calories) per gram, fat being first. It's important to ensure that young people are aware of safe drinking limits and know how to assess the alcoholic strength of products, particularly some of the recently marketed "designer drinks", as these may have a deceptively high alcoholic content.

Practical Advice

The advice given for school-aged children also applies to this age group. Consumption of low fat milk should be encouraged daily. Low fat milk and yoghurts are good snacking foods. Foods rich in iron should be consumed at each of the three main meals and iron-enriched or fortified breakfast cereals may make a significant contribution to the iron intake in this age group. It is worth remembering though that breakfast cereals fortified with iron are almost always the refined processed ones, where manufacturers are obliged by law to fortify because processing removes all the minerals. For example, processing strips wheat of 25 nutrients, but the law only demands that four of them (iron and vitamins B1, B2 and B3) are added back. It's far better if we promote home-made muesli made from jumbo oats, sunflower seeds, nuts and raisins.

Of course, fruit and vegetable consumption should be encouraged daily (at least five portions daily). Consumption of refined or commercially processed foods should be discouraged and whole grain breads, brown rice and brown pasta are better than their white alternatives. High-fat foods, high-sugar foods, and high-salt foods should also be avoided as much as possible, so foods like chocolate and crisps should not be consumed as snacking foods but only as treats.

Binge drinking is a serious problem and is on the increase. Excessive drinking will contribute to liver problems.

Thinness should not be the objective. It should always be health; therefore, physical activity should be encouraged. Let's try to encourage less television and other lifestyle habits that do not promote health.

It our children find it difficult to eat breakfast then try introducing them to smoothies. These are an excellent alternative to solid breakfasts and I have given sample recipes for smoothies in Appendix 5. These smoothies will supply our children with vitamins and minerals (from the fruit and the juice), fibre (from the fruit) and calcium and protein (from the yoghurt).

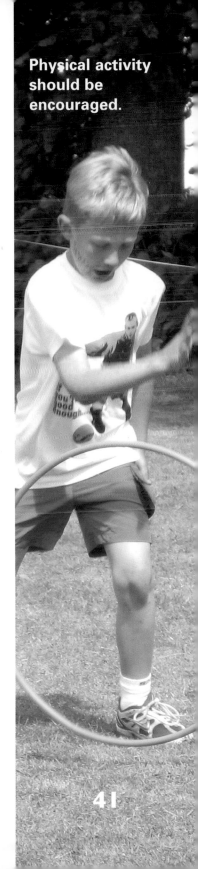

Physical activity should be encouraged.

41

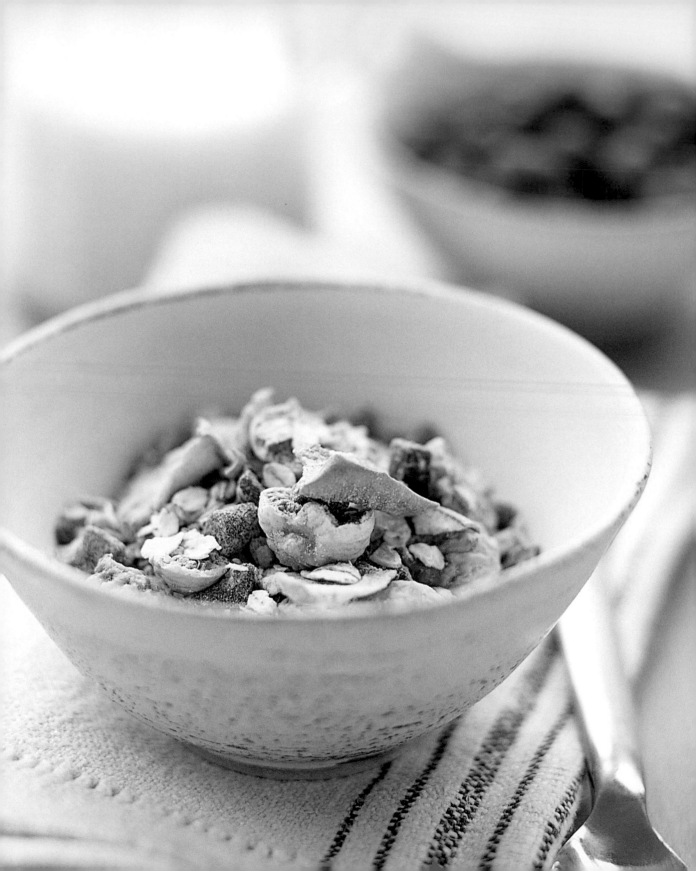

Chapter 6

Healthy Eating –
The Balanced Diet

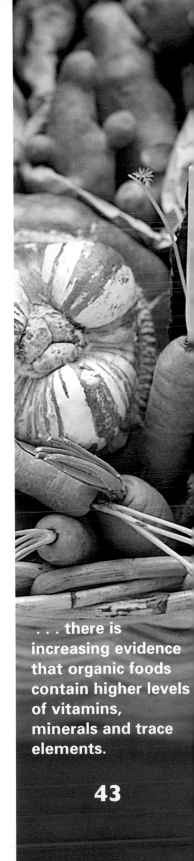

Experts would say that if we consume a balanced diet there is no need for supplementation, and there is currently a great deal of conflicting advice about the use of vitamin and/or mineral supplements. Today's diet has drifted some way off what is considered an ideal intake and balance of nutrients. While it could be argued that little overall change has taken place throughout much of man's history, this cannot be true for the last several decades, when our intakes of saturated fat, sugar and salt have increased while low-glycaemic or slow-release carbohydrates and unsaturated fat intakes have reduced.

There are circumstances when it may be advisable to give our children a supplement. We need to consult our doctor for further advice.

We as consumers are told as long as we consume a balanced diet we will get all the nutrients, and that includes vitamins and minerals, we need But food is not what it used to be. A very useful book by McCance and Widdowson, The Composition of Foods (6th edn, 2002), tells us that there was approximately a 76% decline in the trace mineral content of UK grown fruit and vegetables between 1940 and 1991. That's one of the reasons that we as parents are often advised to give our children vitamin/mineral supplements.

I recommend buying organically grown fruit and vegetables. This is because there is increasing evidence that organic foods contain higher levels of vitamins, minerals and trace elements than do non-organic foods. Organic foods are often more expensive, but greater demand is pushing prices down.

Food production is linked strongly to profit and refining foods makes them last longer so there's more profit to be made. The food industry

. . . there is increasing evidence that organic foods contain higher levels of vitamins, minerals and trace elements.

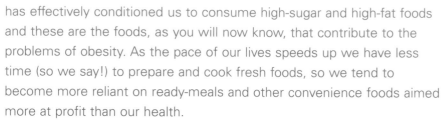

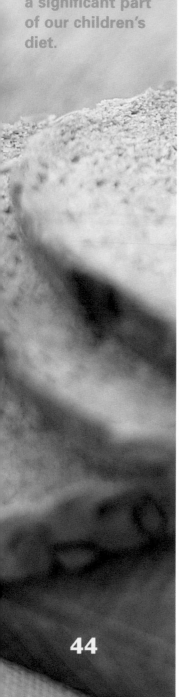

Unprocessed foods are the best choices and should make up a significant part of our children's diet.

has effectively conditioned us to consume high-sugar and high-fat foods and these are the foods, as you will now know, that contribute to the problems of obesity. As the pace of our lives speeds up we have less time (so we say!) to prepare and cook fresh foods, so we tend to become more reliant on ready-meals and other convenience foods aimed more at profit than our health.

The problem is how do we the consumers know whether the foods we consume actually contain the levels of vitamins and minerals that they should contain? Processed foods for example undergo a number of processes between harvesting the raw materials at the farm, to the final product on our plate.

Processing and refining foods strips away the vitamins and minerals from those foods, e.g. the branny outer layers of the unprocessed/refined original food. A good example here is the difference between wholemeal flour and white flour, where most of the B vitamins (and fibre), which are found in the germ of the grain, are removed during the milling process designed to produce white flour.

Therefore, if our children consume a great deal of refined or highly processed foods, with little fruit and vegetables, the chances are that their diet will be low in vitamins and minerals. In such cases, supplementation with a multivitamin/mineral may be advised. Before we put our children on supplements however, we should seek the advice of our doctor or dietitian. In addition, supplementation with vitamins and minerals may also be advised if our children are on a low calorie diet. Again, ask your doctor for advice before giving supplements to your child.

As a guide to healthy eating, carbohydrate-rich foods should provide most of our dietary energy. That said, for optimum health it is important that individuals consume their requirements of protein, fat, water and micronutrients. Therefore, carbohydrate-rich foods that supply significant amounts of other nutrients are valuable. For example, bread, pasta, rice and grain-based foods are a good source of B vitamins. Legumes, meat, fish, nuts, soy products and grain foods are a good source of protein. Fruit and vegetables are a good source of ß-carotenes, some B vitamins and vitamin C. Dairy foods, e.g. yoghurts, are a good source of calcium, protein and riboflavin. Most naturally occurring carbohydrate-rich foods are low in fat and are high in fibre. For a given amount of carbohydrate they give a greater stomach fullness, which will help reduce excessive eating. Examples of foods that contribute to health and examples of those that do not contribute to health (treats only) are given in Figures 6.1 and 6.2.

Examples of foods and drinks children *should* consume often

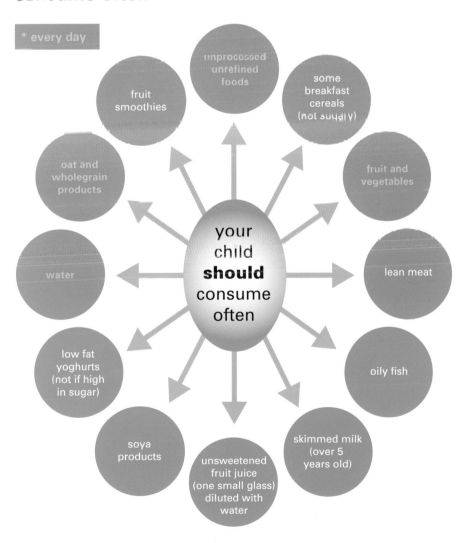

Figure 6.1

Examples of foods and drinks children should consume often

Examples of foods and drinks children *should not* consume often

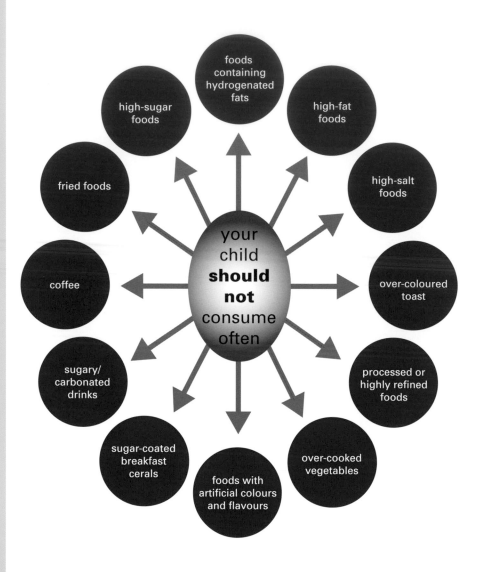

Tips for a Healthy Diet – A Summary

- Eating should be a pleasant aspect of life; we must ensure our children's diet is sustainable, so enjoying food is very important.

- It is important for our children to eat a variety of different foods.

- Don't be afraid to reduce portion sizes, let's ensure our children eat the right amount to be a healthy weight.

- Starchy fibrous foods should be an important part of every diet, so we should encourage our children to eat plenty of foods rich in starch and fibre.

- We must encourage our children to eat plenty of fruit and vegetables, (remember the 5-a-day rule).

- We must ensure our children do not consume too many sugary foods and drinks.

- We need to discourage our children from eating too many fat-rich foods.

- We should try to encourage our children to eat oily fish twice a week.

Alternative Food Choices

Take a look at the following table which gives examples of foods with high energy density (high-fat and/or high-sugar) on the left with some alternatives on the right. Bear in mind that fruit is always an excellent alternative to a number of the products listed on the left even if they are not arrowed as such.

We should not expect to change poor eating habits overnight, we need to take our time. Be patient but persistent. Remember, it's the health of our children that is paramount. Poor dietary habits may not show signs of poor health now, but think long term. Is your children's diet (is your diet) promoting health?

It's a combination of eating more healthily and being physically active that will protect our children from poor health and excess weight gain.

47

Alternatives to high energy density foods

Table 6.1

Alternatives to high energy density foods

Butter or margarine	Low-fat spread, do not use hydrogenated or partially hydrogenated fats
Whole milk and its products	Skimmed or semi-skimmed milk and products made from them, low fat yoghurt, fromage frais
Fried products, e.g. chips	Grilled or baked foods (including oven chips), use a low-fat oil spray
Milk Chocolate	Dark chocolate (70% cocoa solids) which is full of antioxidants, or dried fruit full of minerals and fibre
Sugar coated cereals	Rolled oats (large porridge oats) sweetened with fruit, muesli (read the label to ensure it's not high in salt or sugar), wholegrain cereals, rice flakes or puffed brown rice or Home made muesli made with jumbo oats, nuts, seeds and dried fruit – an excellent start to the day with a glass of juice
Carbonated (gassy) drinks	Water, low calorie squashes, skimmed milk, fruit juice (take care with very young children as fruit juice can contribute to tooth decay). Fruit juice should never be given in babies' bottles.
Cakes and biscuits	Cereal bars (take care – read the labels to ensure no hydrogenated fat), fruit, breakfast cereal with skimmed milk, sandwiches using wholegrain breads with low-fat spread

Chapter 7

Vitamins

Vitamins should not be regarded as a food substitute; they do not supply energy. They are only required in very small amounts to promote health and prevent development of clinical deficiency. They are classified according to their solubility, fat-soluble vitamins (A, D, E and K) and water-soluble vitamins (B-complex and vitamin C). Fruit and vegetables are excellent sources of vitamins; hence it is very important that we consume these food types daily.

To look at individual vitamins and minerals in great detail is beyond the scope of this book. I will however outline some good sources of vitamins and minerals and include some basic information relating to each one.

Vitamin B1 (Thiamin)

This is a member of the B-complex group of vitamins, and is necessary for the functioning of the nervous system. It's easily destroyed by air, water and caffeine. Good sources of thiamin include whole wheat, oatmeal, peanuts, pork, bran, milk and most vegetables. Excess intake of thiamin is removed via the urine. Cooking easily destroys this vitamin, so care must be taken with cooking times and method, e.g. it is often better to steam than to boil. If boiling is necessary I suggest the amount of cooking water is reduced to a minimum to reduce the amount of vitamins lost into the water. Vitamin B1 is often called a 'feel good' vitamin. Lack of this vitamin results in the disease called beriberi.

Vitamin B2 (Riboflavin)

Like the other B vitamins, this vitamin is not stored in the body and must be replaced daily. Good sources include milk, almonds, liver, kidney, cheese, leafy green vegetables, fish, wholemeal bread and eggs. Unlike thiamin, this vitamin is not destroyed by heat. Deficiency may reduce

It's the unprocessed foods such as fruit and vegetables which have the highest levels of vitamins.

49

energy levels, because this vitamin is needed to turn fat, protein and sugar into energy. Insufficient levels also result in cracking of the skin at the corners of the mouth and fissuring of the lips. Large doses of riboflavin (as may be found in vitamin supplements) may result in a yellow discoloration in the urine which is not harmful.

Though vitamins do not supply us with energy, they are important for us to be able to get the energy from our diet

Vitamin B3 (Niacin)

This vitamin is important for normal brain function and has been linked to schizophrenia and depression. Niacin improves skin health, circulation and the digestive system. Good sources of this vitamin include liver, lean meats, peanuts, fish, eggs, sunflower seeds and prunes.

Vitamin B5 (Pantothenic Acid)

This vitamin is involved with the breakdown of all foods, so is involved in energy metabolism. It is widely distributed in animal and plant tissue, and good sources include whole wheat, peas, lentils, eggs, mushrooms and brown rice.

Vitamin B6 (Pyridoxine)

Like the other B vitamins, this vitamin needs to be replaced in our diet daily. This vitamin is required for efficient absorption of vitamin B12. Good sources include brewer's yeast, wheat bran, wheat germ, liver, kidney, heart, cabbage, milk, eggs, brown rice, sunflower seeds and beef. Over-cooking reduces this vitamin in food, so take care with cooking times.

Vitamin B12 (Cobalamin)

This vitamin occurs naturally in almost all animal products, including milk and cheese, and needs calcium for proper absorption in the body. Green

Water soluble vitamins are easily lost from the body and so have to be replaced daily for optimum health.

50

plants do not contain this vitamin. Although we need very little, our absorption is often inadequate, and vegans in particular may need to take supplements. Like vitamin B1, this vitamin is often referred to as a 'feel good' vitamin.

Folic Acid

Folic acid is important for the breakdown of most amino acids (protein), and rich food sources include liver, yeast extract and green leafy vegetables. A diet that is rich in other B vitamins and vitamin C is usually rich in folic acid also.

Biotin (sometimes known as Vitamin H)

Biotin is required for breakdown of glucose, fat and protein. Biotin deficiencies are rare, because only very small amounts are needed daily. Biotin is widely distributed in many foods, including milk, cheese, liver, egg yolks, nuts (peanuts and walnuts), and lentils and is also made by the bacteria found in our intestines.

Vitamin C (Ascorbic Acid)

Vitamin C is an antioxidant, and is an essential water-soluble vitamin. Though plants and most mammals are able to synthesise their own vitamin C, humans cannot. The primary vitamin C deficiency in humans is scurvy. Vitamin C is important for the formation of collagen, in addition it has an important role as an antioxidant against many types of free radical compounds (toxic compounds related to some cancers and ageing, levels of which are significantly increased with smoking or pollution). It is worth noting that vitamin C recycles vitamin E (see below) and in this sense there is synergy between these vitamins. Supplementary vitamin C is thought to decrease the duration of common cold episodes. The best sources of vitamin C are fruit and vegetables, in particular broccoli, sprouts, oranges, strawberries and kiwi fruit. The vitamin is easily destroyed by heat, so raw fruit and vegetables usually have a higher content than their cooked counterparts.

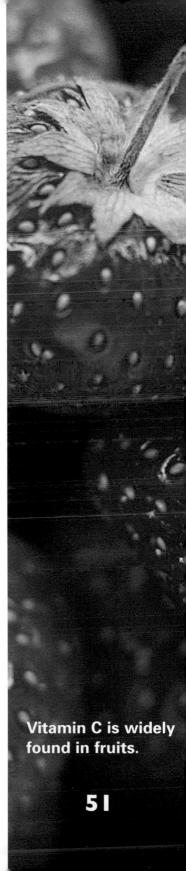

Vitamin C is widely found in fruits.

51

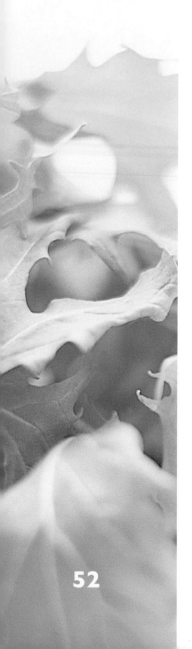

Remember! Essential vitamins are those which are needed to be supplied via the food we eat, our bodies cannot make them.

Vitamin E

Vitamin E is essential for normal function of the immune system, and is one of the most important antioxidants. Unlike vitamin C (another anti-oxidant) which is water soluble, vitamin E is fat soluble. Primary sources of vitamin E include certain vegetable oils, green leafy vegetables, nuts, wheat germ, poultry, fish, fortified breakfast cereals and whole grains.

Vitamin A

Retinol is the common form of vitamin A, but it can also be made in the body from ß-carotene. Like vitamin A, ß-carotene has antioxidant properties. Retinol is an essential component in vision, in fact worsening of night vision is an early sign of vitamin A deficiency. ß-carotene is stored under the skin and is converted to retinol only when needed. Good sources of vitamin A include liver, fish oils and dairy products. However up to one-third of dietary vitamin A comes from ß-carotene, mainly from plant foods, e.g. carrots and other brightly coloured vegetables and fruit. We must not be tempted to give our children vitamin A supplement without consulting a paediatric dietitian first; high levels of this vitamin are toxic.

Vitamin D

This vitamin is important for bone development, and is produced in the body by the influence of sunshine. There are few dietary sources of this vitamin, but it's found in fatty fish, e.g. herring, mackerel, pilchards, sardines and tuna. Other sources include eggs and fortified foods including margarine, some yoghurts and breakfast cereal.

Excessive intake of vitamins and minerals can be harmful to our children, so take care with supplements

Vitamin K

This vitamin is needed for blood clotting properties, and the only major sign of deficiency is defective blood coagulation. Good sources include green leafy vegetables, fruit, dairy produce, vegetable oils, cereals and meats.

Chapter 8

Minerals

Calcium

Calcium forms the main structural component of bone. It is the mineral found in the largest quantity in the body. About 99% of total body calcium is located in the bones, the other 1% is found in blood (necessary for coagulation), muscle and nervous tissue (for muscle contraction and nerve conduction). Inadequate consumption of calcium within the first 30–40 years of life may be associated with increased risk of osteoporosis (a progressive loss of bone mass).

A number of nutrition and lifestyle factors have an impact on the rate of mineral loss from the skeleton. Low levels of physical activity, smoking and alcohol intake are all associated with osteoporosis (weak or brittle bones common in women over the age of 50 years). This is another reason, therefore, that we as loving parents encourage our children to take part in regular physical activity and discourage them from smoking or alcohol abuse when they get older.

Calcium is reported to inhibit the absorption of iron from food, so that these two nutrients should not be taken together in large amounts. Where both iron status and calcium status are in doubt, we must take care with the use of supplements. I suggest we should seek advice from a doctor or paediatric dietician before any supplements are given to our children. Good sources of calcium include bread, dairy products, some canned fish, some vegetables including broccoli and spinach, and some calcium enriched grain products. Calcium is found in good balance with magnesium in nuts and seeds.

Iron

Red meat is an excellent source of iron, as it contains haem which is readily absorbed by our bodies. Fish and poultry also contain haem iron, but not as much as red meat. In contrast, cereals, legumes, whole grains

Nuts and seeds are good sources of calcium. Young children need calcium for strong bones

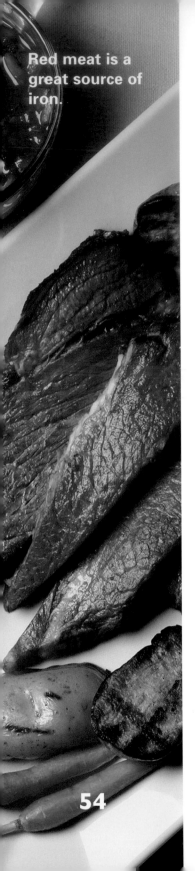

Red meat is a great source of iron.

and deep green leafy vegetables contain non-haem iron, which is not so readily absorbed, but these products are still an important source of this very important mineral. Dried fruits (apricots, prunes, dates), beans, peas, tofu, kale and spinach are iron rich foods that should be consumed by vegetarians. Iron supply can be increased by:

● eating more lean red meat,

● not taking tea or coffee with meals,

● drinking orange juice with breakfast cereal,

● cooking in cast iron cookware,

● frequently eating mixed meals, and

● wisely using iron supplements (consult your doctor first).

Inhibitors of iron absorption include tea, coffee, eggs, cow's milk, wheat bran, soy products and fibre. Avoiding tea or coffee with breakfast and taking vitamin C (orange juice) can triple the amount of iron absorbed from a meal. Eating meals containing a variety of foods is certainly best: for example, eating meat, fish or poultry with vegetables will result in more non-haem iron being absorbed from the vegetables than if the vegetables had been eaten alone.

Unrefined foods are the best sources of both vitamins and minerals.

Magnesium

Magnesium is used as an enzyme co-factor by around 300 different enzyme systems in the body; it's therefore very important for many of the body processes we rely on for health. It's also important for the metabolism of glucose, the regulation of the heart beat and the proper functioning of our muscles. I'm always concerned about bone health in young girls (I have a daughter), so it's worth noting that magnesium is also needed for the absorption of calcium and therefore bone deposition and strength. Good sources of magnesium include whole grain cereals, seeds and legumes. Since most (around 80%) of the magnesium in cereal grains is found in the germ and bran, processed cereal products lose a great deal of their magnesium content during processing or refining. Dairy and meat products provide a moderate amount of magnesium. Deficiency of magnesium shows itself as progressive muscle weakness and failure to thrive.

Zinc

Both animal and human studies have found that zinc deficiency results in a stunting of growth that can be reversed by zinc supplementation. Zinc supplementation may serve as an antioxidant, blocking the increase in free-radical damage, which you will remember results in cancers and premature ageing. Good sources of zinc include animal products such as meat, fish and poultry.

Copper

Symptoms of copper deficiencies in infants and young children include weak bones and increased susceptibility to infections. If the deficiency is prolonged, then anaemia may develop. Good sources of copper include organ meats (especially liver), seafood (especially oysters), nuts and seeds. High levels of vitamin C and dietary zinc will reduce the absorption of copper, and may lead to a reduced copper status.

Chromium

The primary role of chromium is to increase the effects of insulin in stimulating the uptake of glucose, amino acids and triglycerides. Chromium ingestion has been related to several health benefits, e.g. improved glucose tolerance in subjects with poor glucose tolerance. Insufficient chromium could result in an individual developing glucose intolerance and type 2 diabetes. Diets high in simple carbohydrate, e.g. glucose and fructose, will result in reduced chromium levels. Good sources include mushrooms, prunes, nuts, asparagus, and whole grains. When taken with vitamin C absorption of chromium is increased, foods prepared in stainless steel pans etc. can increase the amount of chromium available due to the leaching of chromium from the pans by the action of acid foods.

For the government's recommendations (reference nutrient intakes), for daily intakes of the vitamins and minerals see the chart in Appendix 7 at the back of this book.

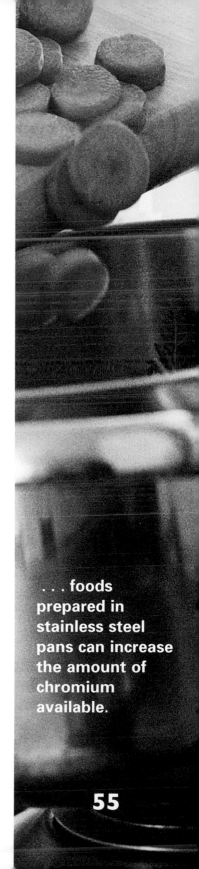

. . . **foods prepared in stainless steel pans can increase the amount of chromium available.**

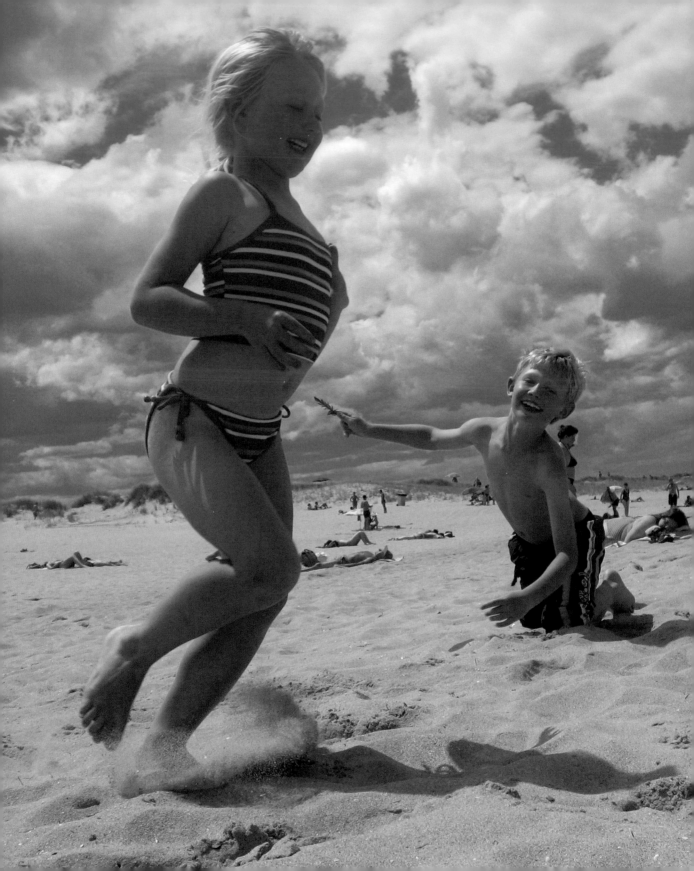

Chapter 9

Physical activity

The link between obesity, heart health and lack of physical activity is very strong. It is possible that our generation of children could be almost free of heart disease simply by taking part in regular physical activity and consumption of wholesome unrefined foods. As parents we need to encourage our children to take part in some sort of activity on a daily basis.

Being more physically active is one of the most important single factors contributing to cardiovascular health, and this is not just because of its relationship to weight loss. Despite this, it's clear that we and our children are becoming much more sedentary, we tend to drive our children everywhere, and we allow them to spend much of their time in front of computers and television. In addition there is a great deal of pressure on making sure they are as academic as possible so that even young children now have large chunks of homework, and often this will reduce the time available to participate in physical activities. If we want our children to be healthy and not over-weight or obese we must encourage more activity; we have to get them moving.

I do not mean that they have to become elite athletes; we need to encourage the simple and enjoyable activities. The important thing is to get them to participate in regular physical activity every day for about one hour. If we as parents or carers could also participate then this would be very helpful. For example at the park give them a run for their money for short distance races, or bike ride together in suitable and safe places. We could even have skipping competitions in the back yard. Apart from burning calories, it's good to remember the heart is a muscle and if it's worked it will become stronger. We only have one heart so let's look after it.

There is no need to count calories. Follow the dietary tips already given in this book, especially the consumption of unrefined foods such as fruit and vegetables.

A combination of eating healthy foods and being physically active will protect our children from poor health.

When trying to keep a healthy weight, being physically active does not mean that our children can consume as much food as they would like. We must realise that if our children burn more calories than they consume they will lose weight. It's important to maintain a degree of control of the types and quantity of foods our children consume. You may remember from what I said earlier in this book that foods high in sugar will result in cravings and increased insulin production, so even if our children are participating in more physical activity we must discourage consumption of these foods types. Always choose the unrefined carbohydrate foods which will give a slower release of their energy. Fruit and vegetables (yes I know I keep repeating myself) should be high on the list of food choices.

Beginning Exercise (child and adult)

Getting started is often the hardest part of becoming more physically active, and, if you are getting on in years, can even be dangerous if you do not take appropriate precautions. We should encourage our children to start slowly and increase the duration and intensity gradually. It makes no sense to put our children off participating in physical activity by rushing things. By the way, if you are over forty years of age and are just getting started yourself, it is important for you to check with your doctor before starting an exercise programme. Some other practical considerations include the following:

- Know your physical limitations.
- Think safety first.
- Choose low impact activities to protect joints.
- Choose an activity that is enjoyable and therefore sustainable.
- Choose a time of day that is convenient.
- Maintain adequate hydration, drink plenty of water.

Type of Exercise for Maximising Health

Endurance exercise is of course what I am talking about, and this involves repetitive movement of the large muscle groups of the body, for

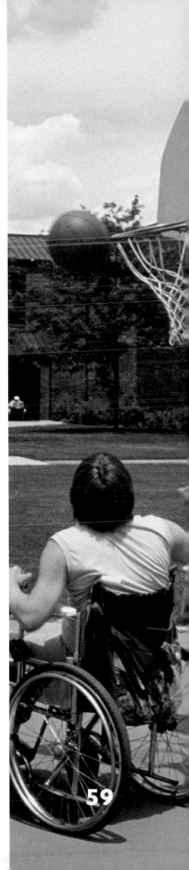

an extended amount of time. Remember our children must have fun and the exercise needs to be sustainable. Good examples include:

- walking
- swimming
- stair-climbers
- elliptical training machines
- skipping
- light jogging
- cycling
- martial arts training
- dynamic yoga classes
- most sports
- **playing!**

The important thing is that anything that gets our children moving is going to work. It may be a good idea to mix up the types of exercise so that they do not get bored; remember the things that are enjoyable are more likely to last.

The Importance of Physical Activity

The benefits of physical activity (exercise) cannot be over-stated. Currently our children are very much less active than we were. There are several reasons for this including spending too much time watching television and playing computer games. In addition, they have less time to play outside due to problems relating to safety etc. and many are not allowed to walk to school, also for reasons of safety. Children therefore burn fewer calories. Couple this with the higher consumption of processed foods and we have a recipe for weight gain and all its associated problems.

Regular appropriate physical activity has been linked with improved health and should be an important part of the overall strategy to control weight. This is even more important as our children get older, and they

59

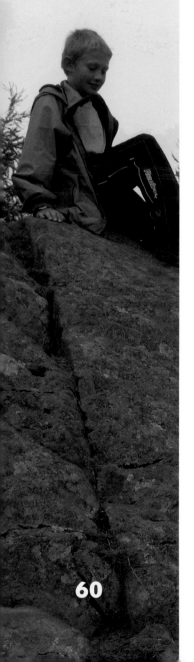

Physical activity releases endorphins, which help us feel happier and more alert.

need to be encouraged to be as active as possible. Being physically active will have an all-round positive effect on health, and apart from the resultant feeling of well being, there are other associated physical benefits. Moderate levels of activity help improve the quality of sleep and help keep bowels working efficiently.

Our metabolic rate is unique to each of us, and this goes some way in explaining why an eating strategy that works for one person may not work for another. Basically the more muscle our children carry (and that also means less fat) the higher will be their metabolic rate. This is because muscle tissue burns or uses fuel taken into the body in the form of food whereas fat tissue does not. Thus, the leaner or more muscular the body, the more food a person will be able to eat without weight gain. Physical activity promotes muscle and reduces fat and at the same time increases metabolic rate.

The good news is that we do not need to be athletic or carry out high intensity physical activity to get real benefits in terms of health and weight control. Walking, cycling and swimming are excellent forms of physical activity if our children do not want to be part of a sports club. Skipping or kicking a ball around the back garden, climbing stairs instead of taking lifts are also excellent forms of exercise.

The point is that we need to encourage increased physical activity and discourage too much television, etc. Interestingly, more body fat is burnt off when intensity is low and when oxygen is used easily. As a guide this means if your child is walking or perhaps jogging, then they need to be able to hold a conversation without struggling. If they cannot talk they are probably working too hard.

Physical activity also releases chemicals in the brain called endorphins; these chemicals help us feel happier and more alert. In addition to endorphins, other chemicals called neurotransmitters are also released which help to suppress appetite.

Another major benefit of being physically active is the improvement in blood circulation and the lowering effect on cholesterol. Remember high levels of blood cholesterol are a risk factor for coronary heart disease.

It just keeps getting better, because in addition to all the above benefits associated with regular physical activity, the chances of our children getting osteoporosis are also reduced. Any physical activity that puts bones under a little stress increases bone density by forcing calcium into them. While the benefits apply to both boys and girls, the greatest benefit will be afforded to girls as they get older. Women reach their peak bone mass (bone strength) by the age of thirty-five years, so it's crucial to build up as much of this as is possible before then. Some good examples of activities that encourage strong bones include jogging, tennis, brisk walking, stair climbing, badminton, and cycling. For parents, activities like housework, carrying shopping and gardening also count.

So inactive children not only increase their chances of gaining weight but they also allow their bone density to reduce, that is, their bones become weaker. We as adults tend to become frailer as we age and some degree of loss of bone strength is inevitable. However, regular physical exercise will reduce this loss in strength. As if all the above benefits are not enough, regular physical activity keeps reflexes sharp and also improves coordination. This in addition to stronger muscles will help protect us from falling and breaking bones as we age.

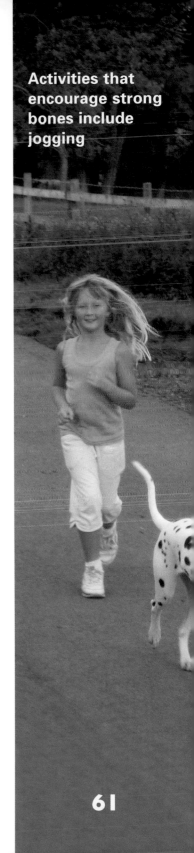

Activities that encourage strong bones include jogging

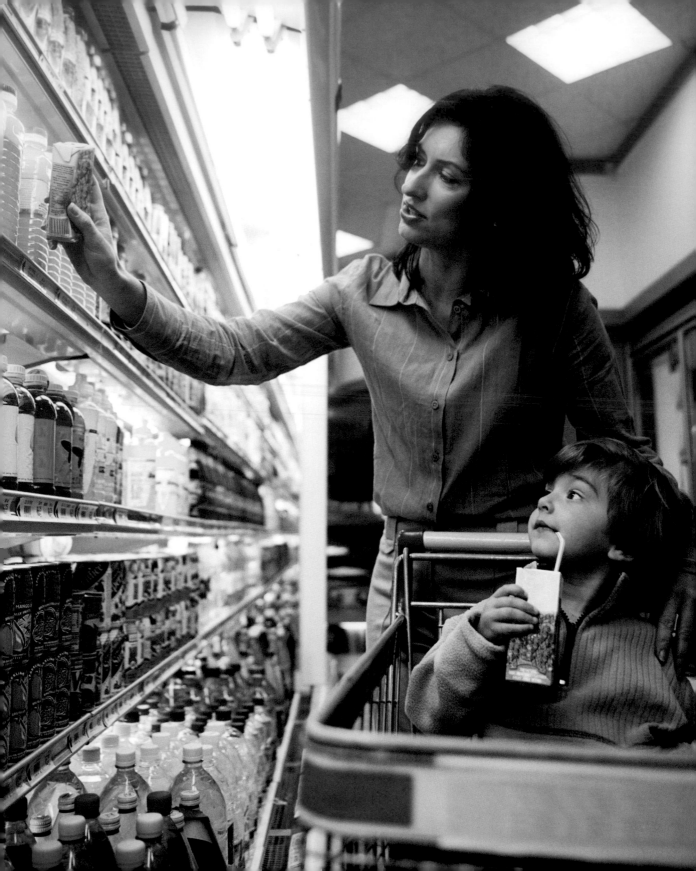

Chapter 10

Reading food labels

We all need to be aware of what's in the foods we consume, and a great deal of this information can be found on the packaging of foods. The problem is that this information can often be confusing and sometimes even misleading. There are foods that have to be sold under prescribed names, and good examples include margarine and ice-cream, which contain specified quantities of ingredients.

Food manufacturing companies are controlled by law as far as nutritional claims, (e.g. low fat) are concerned. Many countries now show nutritional information as well as the list of ingredients that make up the product. Nutrition labels have to show the amount of energy (kcal and kJ), protein, carbohydrate and fat in 100g of the food, which is useful when comparing different brands. The values are also often given per portion size of the food, which is useful when planning healthy meals.

In addition, values for sugar, saturated fat, fibre and sodium are often given, and I have started to see certain foods, e.g. some margarines, where the packaging states trans-fatty acids levels (usually how low levels are in the product). Labels making specific claims have to show values for the nutrient about which the claim is made, e.g. when a claim is made for vitamin enriched you will see vitamin levels on the packaging.

Let's look at an example of the information found on a biscuit product and then I'll highlight some of the important points which you should look for in future. Firstly let's look at the ingredient list then the nutritional information.

Ingredient list

The first ingredient in the list will be the one used in the largest quantity and the ingredient listed last will be the one used in the smallest

It's worthwhile taking the time to read food labels.

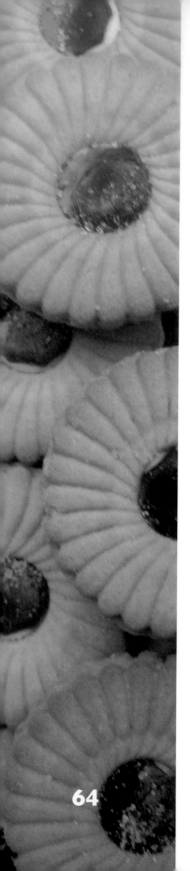

quantity. In other words, the list is given in descending order of quantity (except water). Ingredient lists are useful if you want to compare products for value, or to avoid certain ingredients, e.g. hydrogenated fats. Don't be put off by the thought of reading all those lists. There is no need to read them every time you shop. I found that I was able to identify the healthiest choices very quickly and easily after just a couple of weeks. I thought it a good idea to run through an example:

Ingredients: *Wheat Flour, Blackcurrant Flavour Jam (19%) (containing Glucose Syrup, Sugar Solution, Apples, Humectant (Glycerol), Gelling Agent (Pectin), Citric Acid, Flavouring), Hydrogenated Vegetable Oil, Vegetable Oil, Sugar, Glucose Syrup, Raising Agent (Ammonium Hydrogen Carbonate), Whey Powder, Salt.*

You are also likely to see a note that the product was produced in a factory which handles nuts, and if the product is suitable for vegetarians.

Before I give you the accompanying nutritional information, let's have a look at the ingredient list. Flour is listed first because it is the ingredient used in the largest quantity. Jam is listed second, and you will know having purchased this product that it's a jam biscuit so that should not surprise you. In fact you may be pleased that jam is listed second because it indicates how much jam is used in the biscuit. What follows in brackets after jam is the list of ingredients used to make the jam, and this will tell you something of the quality of the jam, e.g. does it contain high levels of colours and flavours?

Now, the interesting bit of information, as far as health is concerned, is that some of the fat used is hydrogenated. You will recall I highlighted earlier that hydrogenated fat should be avoided as much as is possible because during the process of hydrogenation trans-fats are produced, and these are bad for heart health. Sugar and glucose syrups come next, and these along with the sugars listed in the jam ingredients will tell you the product is going to be high in sugar. If it is, this will show on the nutrition information coming next. The raising agent, whey powder and salt are listed last so

Hydrogenated fats are unhealthy fats and should be avoided. Look for an alternative product

these should be used in small quantities, again confirmed by the nutrition information. However, as I have already pointed out we typically consume around twice the salt we should consume so this is perhaps another reason to find an alternative product – they are out there!

Nutritional information

Now let's look at the nutritional information that will be given on the same packaging for this product. This will often be given in the form of a table, such as the one below

Typical Values	Per 100 g	Per Biscuit
Energy	187.7kJ	335 kJ
	44.6 kcal	80 kcal
Protein	4.8 g	0.9 g
Carbohydrate	69 g	13 g
of which:Sugars	33 g	6.2 g
Fat	17 g	3.2 g
of which: Saturates	14.6 g	2.7 g
Fibre	0.9 g	0.16 g
Sodium	0.2 g	Trace

Table 10.1

Nutritional information

The first thing listed is the energy value for this product. This is 80kcal per biscuit, which should not surprise you, as biscuits are typically energy dense. Biscuits are a good example of foods that are high in both fat and sugar. How much sugar? Well look at the level per 100g of product – carbohydrate makes up 69g. That is 69% of the biscuit is carbohydrate. Now of this, sugar (remember this is a simple carbohydrate) is 33g, that is 33% or one-third of the biscuit is sugar. Think about that, if our children eat three of these then one will be the equivalent of pure sugar.

Now what about the fat? As we have already seen on the ingredient list, some of this is hydrogenated and a glance at the above table will show that just under 15% (14.6%) of the biscuit is saturated fat, and that is not health-promoting. The difference between total fat (17g per 100g of product) and saturated fat (14.6g per 100g of product) is 2.4g per 100g of product, and is likely to be a mix of mono- and poly-unsaturated fats.

The table shows a low level of fibre and it contains sodium (part of salt) and again, we need to reduce our salt levels. When you see sodium listed (but not salt) you can easily work out the equivalent salt level by multiplying the sodium figure by 2.5. So in the biscuit example given earlier, the sodium level was 0.2g per 100g of biscuit. The equivalent salt level is therefore 0.2 g x 2.5 = 0.5g per 100g of product.

To help clarify what this level of salt means, a little salt means no more than 0.3g of salt per 100g of product and a lot of salt would be 1g per 100g of product. The example I have given above falls between the two.

Nutritional Claims

Voluntary guidelines are in place in order to govern the meaning of some nutrition claims. However, claims can be quite misleading, for example if a claim of reduced fat (or sugar) is made, then that product must contain 25% less fat (or sugar) than the original or standard product. Use the following as a guide.

Biscuits are typically high in energy but low in nutrients

Table 10.2
Nutritional claims

Claim	Meaning (per100g food)	Claim	Meaning (per 100g of food)
Low fat	No more than 5g	Low sodium	No more than 40mg
Low sugar	No more than 5g	Saturates free	No more than 0.1g
Low saturates	No more than 3g	High fibre	More than 6g

When a label states 'no added sugar', it means that no sugars or any ingredient (e.g. fruits or fruit concentrates) composed mainly of sugars should be added to the food. In addition, there are a number of claims made by food manufacturers that are not covered by voluntary government guidelines. These claims may mean different things to different people, so you will need to read the ingredient list and nutrition information with care. Such claims include the following examples:

'Virtually fat free' means that there will be very little fat in the product. When a label boasts 90% fat free, remember that it contains 10% fat, and this does not mean virtually fat free.

'Lower fat' usually means the product will contain less fat than the standard product on which it is based. To find out how much lower, you will need to read the nutrition information. The chances are that the level of fat is not a great deal lower, otherwise the manufacturers would be claiming low fat or reduced fat.

'Half fat' simply means the food contains half the fat of its standard product counterpart.

'Light' or **'lite'** is a difficult one. It could mean light in weight, light in colour or more often light in fat.

So what about diet products? Well, according to the food labelling regulations the word 'diet' can only be used on products that make a low calorie claim. This means delivering no more than 40 calories per 100g, or in the case of a drink 100ml, or if a serving is typically less than 100g then the claim should apply to the serving size. The claim must be accompanied by the statement '. . . can help slimming or weight control only as part of a calorie controlled diet'.

The weight of the food in the packet or tin is usually given on the food label accompanied by a big letter 'e'. This means that the average quantity (taken from a number of packets or tins) of food must be accurate, but that the weight on each packet or tin may vary slightly.

The Food Standards Agency Traffic Light System

The Food Standards Agency (FSA) introduced this system in an attempt to clarify some of the difficulties or confusion when buying foods. The traffic light scheme is designed to provide at-a-glance information on whether a food is high, medium or low in total fat, saturated fat, sugar and salt. Simply, we are advised to buy, and therefore consume, less of

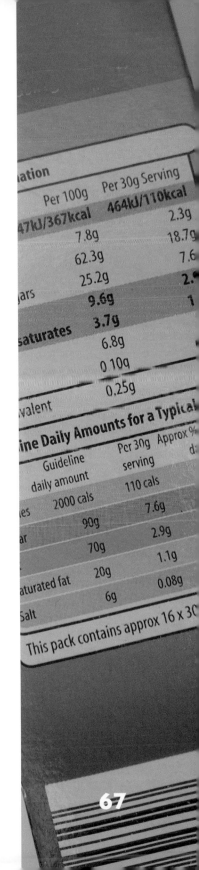

the foods highlighted by the red light and more of the foods highlighted by the green light, see Figure 10.1.

Figure 10.1

Traffic light system

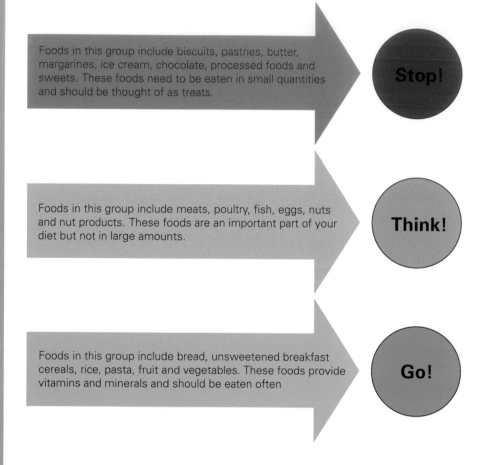

Foods in this group include biscuits, pastries, butter, margarines, ice cream, chocolate, processed foods and sweets. These foods need to be eaten in small quantities and should be thought of as treats.

Stop!

Foods in this group include meats, poultry, fish, eggs, nuts and nut products. These foods are an important part of your diet but not in large amounts.

Think!

Foods in this group include bread, unsweetened breakfast cereals, rice, pasta, fruit and vegetables. These foods provide vitamins and minerals and should be eaten often

Go!

Sainsbury, Asda and Waitrose, the Co-op and Marks and Spencer have all opted for a traffic-light label. However, the Food and Drinks Federation introduced Guideline Daily Amounts (GDA's) in an attempt to take the guesswork out of what we should be eating and thus make planning a healthier diet easier. Several food retailers have opted for this system over the FSA's Traffic Light System, believing it's easier for the consumer to understand. The system works by taking the recommended average daily amounts of the following: energy (calories), sugar, fat, saturates and salt.

Reading food labels

To make it easier, they quote the GDA for adult women on food packaging; remember that men and children have different requirements so this system is a guide only. The system identifies these GDAs as shown below.

	Guideline Daily Amount
Energy (Calories)	2000 Calories
Sugar	90g
Fat	70g
Saturates	20g
Salt	6g

Table 10.3

Guideline Daily Amounts (GDAs)

What you see on the packaging is the percentage of the above delivered by the food inside the packet e.g. if the number of calories in the product is 770 then this would be shown as 38.5%. Remember, the figures given are for adults only. For your information, I have given the GDAs for women, men and children (aged 5–10 years) in the following table.

	Calories	Sugar (g)	Fat (g)	Saturates (g)	Salt (g)
Women	2000	90	70	20	6
Men	2500	120	95	30	6
Children (5–10 years)	1800	85	70	20	4

Table 10.4

Guideline Daily Amounts for men, women and children (aged 5–10 years)

Remember!
These are guidelines only, they are not a target

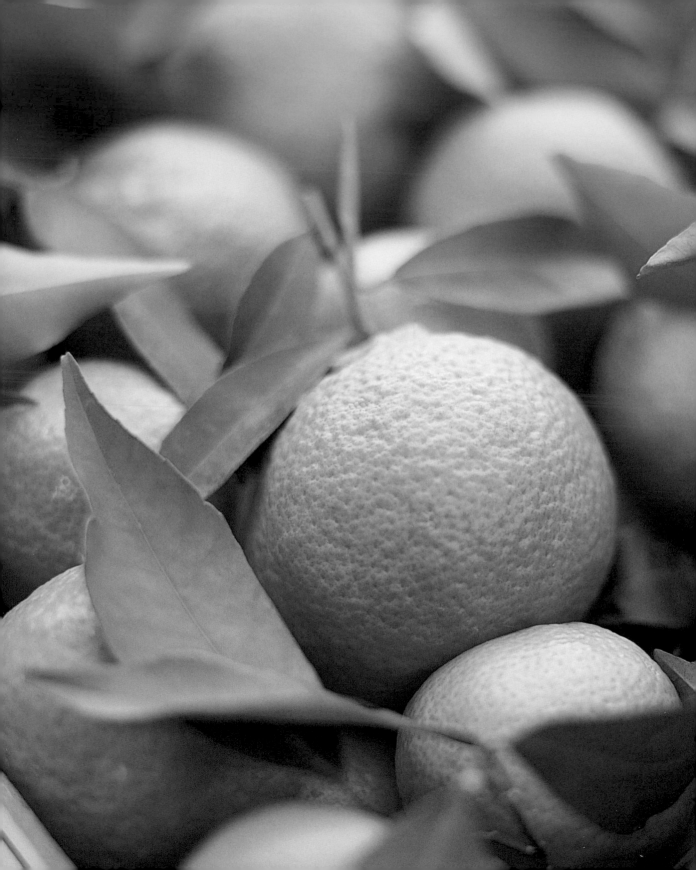

Chapter 11

Diabetes – Some Basics

This disease, which is on the increase, is the inability of the body to control levels of sugar (glucose) in the blood, and carbohydrate has always played a role in its management. There are two main types of diabetes, type 1 and type 2, the latter being the most common.

Type 1 diabetes (previously known as 'juvenile onset or insulin-dependent' diabetes) usually appears during childhood, teenage years or early adulthood. Type 1 diabetics do not have the ability to produce insulin.

Type 2 diabetes (previously known as 'maturity onset or non-insulin-dependent' diabetes) tends to develop after the age of 40 years. Type 2 diabetics have the ability to produce insulin, but in insufficient amounts or they are resistant to the action of insulin.

As parents, I think it's worth considering the very important role that good nutrition and regular physical activity play in preventing type 2 diabetes. I also believe it's worth emphasising here that the most important reason a diabetic needs to control blood sugar levels is to reduce the risk of complications of diabetes, e.g. loss of sight, and not just to lose weight.

Before the advent of insulin therapy the only method of treating type 1 diabetes was by total restriction of carbohydrate from the diet. Carbohydrate restriction played a role through most of the twentieth century. In the early 1980s, the first set of dietary guidelines for people with diabetes recommended that carbohydrate should form 50% of dietary energy, and this carbohydrate should be unrefined.

The messages from research into diabetes to improve quality of life are simple. Glycaemic control (more about this later) is important, and this means consumption of foods with a low glycaemic index so that insulin spikes are not experienced. The largest cause of mortality in the diabetic population is heart disease, and dietary advice needs to reflect this. As

Low glycaemic foods (unrefined foods) release their sugar slowly, so our children will feel fuller for longer.

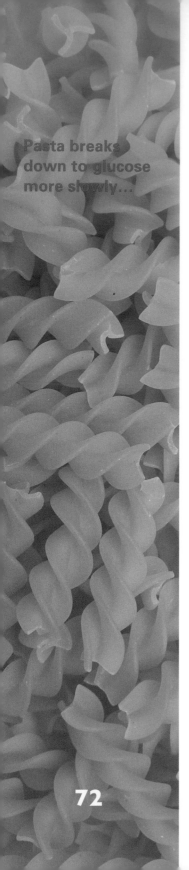

Pasta breaks down to glucose more slowly...

carbohydrate contributes to a large percentage of total energy intake, it is important to know how different carbohydrate-rich foods may influence the health of our children.

Carbohydrates range from the very fast release such as glucose, to the slower release such as starch. They have different properties depending on processing (e.g. refining) both by the food manufacturer and during cooking at home, and their ease of digestion in the body varies. Remember, a given weight of carbohydrate from two different foods can give large differences in glycaemic response. For example, bread will break down quickly to glucose and give a very rapid insulin response, whereas pasta breaks down to glucose more slowly and gives a slower response in terms of insulin production after consumption.

Some Basics about the Glycaemic Index of Foods, and the Link with Diabetes

The organ responsible for the production of the hormone insulin is the pancreas, which is found near the stomach. Insulin does two things really well.

1. It controls the levels of blood glucose.

2. It inhibits the breakdown of body fat to glucose (by inhibiting another hormone also produced by the pancreas, called glucagon, which likes to break down fat). So high blood levels of insulin really slow down the breakdown of body fat, making it more difficult to lose weight.

This is the result of the times when our ancestors were hunter-gatherers, they often experienced times of feast and famine, so that when food was in plentiful supply the body stored it for times when food was scarce. Insulin was the important factor in this process, both helping to accumulate fat and then controlling its depletion. Easy so far isn't it, so why is it that we easily accumulate fat and can find it difficult to reduce it?

Well our digestive systems have taken many thousands of years to evolve, but are expected to cope with our modern foods in 'the blink of an eye' in evolutionary terms. We no longer have to hunt for food

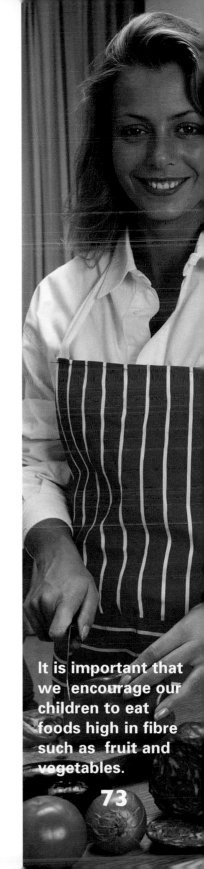

because it's in plentiful supply. In addition, much of today's food is highly processed and therefore is very easily digested; yes, we're back to the insulin spike. As if this was not enough, we no longer need to burn energy finding our food or keeping ourselves warm, as our ancestors had to do.

It is important to maintain low insulin levels when weight gain is an important consideration

Because insulin is key to storing glucose and keeping fat cells intact, it goes without saying that it is very important to maintain low insulin levels when weight loss is the aim. This means we must consume low-GI foods. However take care because this is not the whole story.

The fact that a food has a low GI does not necessarily mean that it is a desirable food; its GI is only one factor to consider when concerned about weight. The other is calorie content of the food. So, it's the combination of low glycaemic index foods with few calories, i.e. low in fat and sugar (surprise surprise) that we should look out for. Dietary carbohydrates, more than any other food, stimulate the pancreas and insulin is released into the blood.

If it takes time to break the food down, for example if the food is less- or un-processed (e.g. whole grains, oats, beans and brown rice) then the pancreas does not have to work too hard because only slow and low levels of insulin release are needed. If on the other hand the diet is consistently high in processed or sugary foods then glucose is quickly released into the blood, and a speedy release of high levels of insulin is needed. Under these circumstances genetically susceptible individuals may have an increased risk of type 2 diabetes.

Eating patterns over the last few decades have resulted in much of our diet being made up of processed foods, i.e. foods where much of the roughage or fibre has been removed. The presence of fibre is responsible for slowing down digestion, hence reducing the need for rapid and high levels of insulin secretion. Therefore, without this fibre, food is more easily broken down, sugars are quickly released and the pancreas has to work harder. Put simply, our new way of preparing and consuming foods means higher blood sugar levels following a meal.

It is important that we encourage our children to eat foods high in fibre such as fruit and vegetables.

73

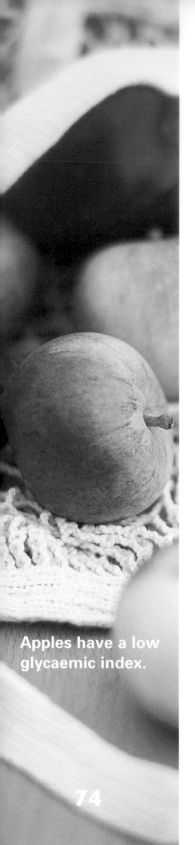

Apples have a low glycaemic index.

Quite apart from the fact that diabetes is promoted in our modern diets, other diseases, notably heart disease, are also promoted.

Insulin also influences the way we break down (metabolise) our foods, and determines whether we burn fat or carbohydrate in order to meet our energy needs. Ultimately, therefore insulin influences the storage of fat as adipose tissue in our bodies. Clearly, it would be of great advantage if we, the consumers, had a way of knowing how to identify foods which produce a rapid response of insulin and foods which produce a slow response. In this way we could effectively reduce our risk of type 2 diabetes. Fortunately, we do have a way of identifying such foods and it's called (you guessed it) the "glycaemic index" of foods.

The glycaemic index has been developed in order to list foods based on what is called their glycaemic response, which means how quickly a food releases glucose into the blood when it's consumed. Those foods which are broken down quickly have the highest glycaemic index, and glucose is given the value of 100. Foods releasing glucose into the blood slowly, e.g. apples, are given a lower glycaemic index (see Appendix 3).

The gradual rise in blood sugar resulting from its slow release from low-GI foods is of significant importance for many people, especially those already suffering from diabetes. The slow release of insulin following low glycaemic foods reduces the risk of heart disease, diabetes and obesity. In this way, low-GI foods benefit people with and without diabetes.

Another way of identifying foods in terms of glucose response is by their glycaemic load, which gives an indication of the amount of sugars a food contains. The glycaemic load is defined as the glycaemic index of a food multiplied by the grams of carbohydrate in a serving, divided by 100. The GI applies to carbohydrates; proteins and fats have no effect on blood glucose, so the proportion of protein and/or fat in a meal has an influence on the glycaemic load. Foods with a low glycaemic loading are more health-promoting than those with a high glycaemic loading.

To summarise, foods with a low GI promote health because they cause lower insulin levels, which helps in fat reduction and helps to reduce blood fat levels. They reduce the temptation to over-eat because they are more satisfying, and reduce the risk of developing diabetes and heart disease.

Food manufacturers often alter the starch granules by heating them in water, which causes the starch to thicken (called gelatinise). We often do this at home, e.g. when we make custard, we heat cornflour (or custard powder) in milk, which then thickens; the same thing happens when we make gravy from flour and water etc. Cornflour and wheat flour are both starchy materials. Starchy foods processed in this way have a higher GI than the original starchy material. This is one of the reasons why processed foods have a higher GI (don't forget another reason is the removal of fibre during the processing of many foods).

Vegetables are a really good source of carbohydrate; we can eat most vegetables because they have a low GI. Most are so low that they have a very small effect on blood sugar levels but still provide us with valuable amounts of vitamins, minerals and fibre. This book does not cover the glycaemic index of all foods. There are many published books where more detail can be found, e.g. *The GI Diet* by Rick Gallop. However, some examples can be found in Appendix 3.

Good low-fat high-carbohydrate choices include:

- Cereal grains, including oats, brown rice, wheat, barley, rye and the products made from them. Breads that are low GI include soya & linseed, granary and pumpernickel

- Fruits, including apples, oranges, dried apricots, bananas, grapes and peaches

- Vegetables, including corn

- Legumes (peas and beans), including baked beans, lentils and kidney beans.

In addition, milk is not only a good source of carbohydrate, but also a source of calcium which is very important for bone health. Adults and children over five years are advised to use skimmed milk and low fat yoghurts to minimise fat intake, but children under the age of five years should not be fed skimmed milk; instead they need full-fat milk.

So let's now focus on the reason why diabetes is linked to heart trouble. It starts with the expanding waist line as we get fatter. As our fat cells

Highly refined foods will have a higher glycaemic index than those foods that are unrefined.

75

get bigger, insulin has trouble attaching to them and therefore is unable to function effectively. Hence, in over-weight and obese people the sugar and fat levels in the blood rise higher than they really should.

When the insulin produced by the pancreas is not working properly it takes much longer than it should to store the fat consumed. This delay results in the depositing of fat and cholesterol in the blood vessels of the heart, hence the link between obesity and heart disease. The carbohydrate or sugars themselves do not cause the heart attack but they create the conditions that lead to one. In addition, obesity itself does not damage the cardiovascular system, but it's an excellent indicator that there is likely to be an unhealthy blood profile. This unhealthy blood profile is more than likely going to reduce your health and maybe even your lifespan.

This brings me right back to the need for regular and appropriate levels of physical activity. The bottom line is that most of us are less active today than our parents and grandparents were. Our food is more refined and we rely more and more on convenience foods which have undergone high levels of processing, which means our digestive systems have to work less hard to break the food down. By now you will see the picture emerging quite clearly I'm sure.

Quite alarmingly, the move towards healthier eating has, in some circumstances, brought us closer to the unhealthy state described in the paragraphs above. To see what I mean, next time you go shopping have a close look at some food labels. Examine the nutritional information on some products described as 'low-fat'. You may be surprised to find that in many cases the fat has been replaced with processed carbohydrates, i.e. lower in fat but very high in sugars – so take care!

At the risk of boring you, let me once more emphasise why we need to control our children's weight. It has little to do with thinness and everything to do with health. I know and understand why being thin is important to many people, e.g. clothes are easier to buy because more clothes are designed for thin people than for larger people; in addition some people associate thinness with beauty. But much more important is what's going on inside our children's bodies. What problems are we storing up for them in later life? This is what should be more important.

Just because a product is sold as lower in fat does not mean it is better for you.

Looking good on the outside is important, but having physically fit blood vessels and a healthy blood chemistry is much more important. Our children (and ourselves) can have both by eating health-promoting foods and being physically active.

I hope your journey through this book has been enjoyable, rewarding and enlightening. It's certainly been an enjoyable experience for me, so until next time, enjoy life, promote health and keep active.

Chapter 12

Frequently Asked Questions

Q What foods are suitable for my child to take to school to snack on?

A Fromage frais, low fat yoghurts, fruit, and some cereal bars are very good. With cereal bars read the label, if they contain high levels of fat, sugar or salt don't buy them. In addition look for hydrogenated or partially hydrogenated fat on the ingredient list, if these fats are present put them back on the shelf.

Q What fruits are the best?

A All fruits are good, but the brightly coloured fruits or fruits where the colour goes right through like strawberries are very good because these will be high in phytochemicals which help protect against a number of diseases. It's a good idea to vary the types of fruit you or your children consume, that way you reduce boredom and increase the chances of consuming a wide spectrum of vitamins, minerals and fibre.

Q Could you explain why saturated fats are not good fats?

A Saturated fats increase blood levels of cholesterol, and high levels of cholesterol are a risk factor for coronary heart disease.

Q Why are omega-3 fats good fats?

A Because they promote a healthy heart and blood vessels, therefore reducing the chance of heart disease later in life. There is also evidence that these fats promote increased mental performance in children.

Q Why do processed foods need to be limited in my child's diet?

A When we consume unrefined or unprocessed foods, it takes our digestive system a long time to break down the food so the release of sugar into the bloodstream is slow and the amount of sugars released is low. This means we do not need to generate high levels of insulin quickly to deal with high sugar levels. Consumption of processed foods means the body breaks down the food quickly during digestion. This means high levels of sugar are released quickly, so the pancreas needs to produce a lot of insulin quickly to control blood levels of the released sugar. It's not a good thing to have high levels of insulin in the blood; insulin is often referred to as the fat-storage hormone and in individuals who are inactive this can lead to excess weight gain.

Q I've been told by a number of people that potatoes are a bad food. Is this true?

A No, potatoes which are boiled or baked with their jackets are OK. Often it's the amount of butter or cream that's added that is the problem. In addition, the worst thing to do with potatoes is to fry them. Fried foods are a problem for a number of reasons, one of which is the fat used. Potatoes are high GI, new potatoes and sweet potatoes are lower GI alternatives. Remember though that potatoes are not to be included in the 5-a-day rule for the consumption of fruit and vegetables.

Q Is it healthier to use butter or margarine?

A This will depend on the margarine. Hydrogenated or partially hydrogenated margarines are particularly bad and in this case butter is the better option. However, there are margarines now readily available which are not hydrogenated and are made from olive oil (rich in unsaturated fats) and these margarines are better than butter, which is of animal origin and is high in saturated fatty acids. All fats solid at room temperature should be used sparingly.

Q Can we exercise too much?

A Yes, for example very young female gymnasts who have over-exercised have been reported to have reduced periods. Most of us however do not approach this level of exercise, so too little exercise or physical activity is a more serious problem.

Q Is it appropriate for very young children to train with weights?

A No, the bones of young children are soft, so training with weights may result in deformation of those bones. If your child wants to train with weights you should seek advice from qualified experts and they should ensure only light weights are used.

Q What is meant by saturated fats and where do they come from?

A These fats are typically animal in origin but some tropical oils also contain saturated fats, e.g. palm oil and coconut oil. Basically saturated fats are hard while unsaturated fats are soft (oils). The fat manufacturers can easily modify unsaturated fats by a process called hydrogenation, to make the fat harder. Hydrogenation therefore converts an oil to a fat and in doing so increases its shelf life and usefulness to the food manufacturer. Remember, we need to avoid hydrogenated or partially hydrogenated fats.

Q Should I stop my children from eating cakes and biscuits?

A No, simply limit when they can eat these foods. They need to be thought of as treats, and eaten perhaps once a week instead of daily. Try to find cakes and biscuits which do not contain hydrogenated or partially hydrogenated fats. Remember it's not just about your child's weight; it's about the promotion of their health.

Q Are organic fruits better for us than normally grown fruits?

A Organically grown fruits should be free of insecticides etc. so from that point of view they are better because they do not deliver those toxins to us, the consumer. Many people also claim that organically grown fruit tastes better and that might be a consideration when encouraging your children to eat more.

Q Are all breakfast cereals good for children?

A No, avoid those coated in sugar or with added sugar or salt. One of the best breakfast cereals is porridge oats, which takes time to be digested and therefore staves off hunger for longer. In addition oats contain both soluble and insoluble fibre. Remember soluble fibre helps control blood cholesterol while the insoluble fibre helps maintain a healthy gut.

Q Should I give my two-year-old daughter skimmed milk?

A No, children under five years should be given full cream milk unless you have been advised otherwise by your doctor.

Q Why are fried foods so bad for us?

A There are a number of reasons. Fried foods by definition are likely to carry more calories than the same food which has been baked, boiled or grilled. In addition frying results in the production of free radicals. Free radicals enable cholesterol to do its damage to our blood vessels and can promote heart disease, cancers and premature aging. By the way, if you use a polyunsaturated fat to fry with, you convert a good fat to a bad fat by converting a cis fat to a trans fat. I know this is more fat chemistry, but trans fats are particularly bad for our health.

Q Should I allow my child to eat crisps?

A Yes, but only as a very occasional treat. Crisps are a food high in fat and salt, and of course they are a fried food. Typically children tend to eat far too many crisps as they are often given as part of a lunch box. This is a habit that needs to be stopped, remember 'treat only'.

Q I have been told that if I put my child on a low or no carbohydrate diet she will lose weight very quickly. Is such a diet a good idea?

A First, let me say that putting our children on diets is not a good idea. As far as the specific question is concerned, any diet that does not include fruit, vegetables and unrefined cereal grain products should be avoided. Remember losing weight per se is not the main aim, it's losing body fat and promoting optimum health. Optimum health will not be the outcome if vitamins and minerals are not delivered in the foods we or our children consume. What you need to reduce, as far as carbohydrates are concerned, are of course the simple carbohydrates, the sweeter sugary foods that will generate high levels of insulin production.

Q I have been told that if I eat a balanced diet I will not need to take supplements, what do you think?

A In general, a diet rich in fruit, vegetables and other unrefined/unprocessed foods will deliver the vitamins and minerals needed on a daily basis. That said, take care when you cook foods because this may result in destruction of many of the vitamins. Remember, the best way for you or your child to get your vitamins and minerals is when they are a part of a whole food. For example, get your vitamin C from fruit and not pills, because the fruit will also give you fibre and other nutrients.

Q What do you think of vitamin and mineral supplements?

A Before I give you my view on supplements, let me first say that the best way of getting vitamins and minerals is as part of a whole food. Basically that means healthy eating. However, that said, many of the foods we consume are processed and refined, and often that means the vitamins and minerals have been stripped away. In addition, we often over-cook foods at home and this destroys vitamins especially vitamins that are water-soluble like vitamin C. If you rely heavily on processed foods, it may be worth considering supplementation. I would suggest a good general multivitamin and mineral, but you should discuss this with your doctor first. In addition, if fish is not a regular part of your and your child's diet, you may like to consider taking EPA fish oil capsules; these are rich in omega-3 fatty acids which are good for heart health.

Q I noticed that you tend not to use the word 'exercise', but instead you talk of physical activity. What's wrong with exercise?

A The reason I tend not to use the word 'exercise' is simply because to many people it conjures up images of expensive gym membership, or performing hard sweaty work which is neither enjoyable nor sustainable. Exercise may also imply something more formal and regimented. Physical activity on the other hand covers a wider range of behaviour. It includes, for example, walking to the shops instead of taking the car, climbing stairs instead of taking the lift or perhaps even walking the dog a little further than normal. These are simple activities that need not cost anything in terms of money or even significant amounts of time. These activities are also more likely to be more enjoyable and sustainable and reduce the chances of us becoming couch potatoes. Being physically active is the important thing when it comes to our health and not necessarily exercising.

Q If you had to suggest one breakfast cereal that was health-promoting, which one would it be and why?

A Without doubt the one I would suggest every time is the large rolled oat cereal suitable for making porridge. Don't be tempted to buy the varieties sold as instant, because these have been processed to enable them to cook out much more quickly. As to the second part of this question, oats contain two types of fibre, soluble, which is good at reducing cholesterol, and insoluble, which is good at promoting gut health. The larger oats also take longer to digest so that hunger is staved off for longer, reducing chances of cravings. As well as being used for porridge, oat cereal can be mixed with dried fruit and fruit juice and eaten as is.

Q When I give my child a meal, I feel it's very important that he eats it all. Don't you think that this is important?

A If you are giving your child portion sizes which are too big, then no I do not think it's important that everything on the plate is eaten. When your child has eaten enough they know it, they have a good feel for when they are full. Instructing them to eat more is a little like force feeding and effectively trains them to eat excess amounts as they grow older; in other words they will put weight on. It's far better to give children smaller portions and let them ask for more if they want more. That said, it is important to monitor what your child eats. Children may not finish a meal for a number of reasons, e.g. they may want to play, or may be in a faddy eating phase. Also they may eat only selected parts of the meal, say potatoes but not sprouts. Monitor but don't force feed.

Q You said in your presentation that a diet high in fruit, vegetables and unrefined cereal grains is best if the diet is high in water also. What do you mean by that?

A These foods are high in fibre, which does its magic by keeping stools soft so that constipation is prevented. The fibre does this by absorbing water from the body, so insufficient water in the diet may result in dehydration. Drinking extra water, and by that I mean something like 8–10 glasses a day, will supply the extra water needed by the fibre and so prevent dehydration.

Q I give my child a vitamin pill every day, but have noticed that his urine is quite yellow in colour. What is causing this?

A The vitamin pills contain riboflavin, a B vitamin, and this is the cause of the colour of your child's urine. Don't be alarmed; this is   .

Q What is a non-essential nutrient?

A This is a nutrient that isn't needed in the diet because the body is able to make it from other nutrients. This is in contrast to an essential nutrient, e.g. vitamin C, where the body is unable to make it from other nutrients, so it needs to be taken in as part of our diet.

Q You have already stated that one of the functions of carbohydrate is for energy. Do carbohydrates have other functions?

A Yes, other functions of carbohydrates include:

● conserving protein during energy production,

● helping to burn fats more efficiently and completely,

● aiding in the normal functioning of the bowel, by providing fibre.

Q You speak of glucose as triggering insulin production and you have said that glucose is a simple sugar. What about fructose, which you have also said is a simple sugar?

A Fructose is converted to glucose in the liver. The liver then releases this glucose into the bloodstream where its level is controlled with insulin. Thus fructose takes longer to get into the blood as glucose and that is why its glycaemic index is lower than glucose.

Q It's good to have a guide as to how much sugar we should be consuming, and you have said that it should be no more than 7% of our energy needs. How much would that be in terms of weight?

A Let's assume you need 2500kcal per day. Sugar is a carbohydrate, and as I have already said, carbohydrates contain 3.75–4kcal of energy per gram. For the sake of making the calculation simple we'll round this up to 4kcal per gram. With this information it's relatively easy to calculate your limit. We should not consume more than 7%, so 7% of 2500kcal is 175kcal. Now all we have to do is divide the 175kcal by 4 kcal to give the weight of sugar in grams. So in this example, the answer will be 175/4 = 43g, which is equivalent to just under 2 ounces. Not much sugar is it? Currently we typically consume more than double this.

Q What is cholesterol?

A Cholesterol is a fat-like substance that is made in the liver. The liver also filters out excess cholesterol to eliminate fat from the body. Cholesterol is also a component of foods we eat, occurring naturally in all animal products. High levels of cholesterol in the blood may lead to heart disease.

84

Q What exactly are invisible fats?

A These are the fats that you cannot see, but are present (often in high levels) in a number of foods. For example the fat you spread on bread will not be covered by the term but the fat found in a biscuit will be. Cakes and biscuits are good examples of foods high in invisible fats.

Q Is chocolate all bad, that is, does chocolate have any good qualities in terms of nutrition?

A No, chocolate isn't all bad, but it needs to be thought of as a treat food and not be an important part of your overall diet. Let's take milk chocolate as an example. Milk chocolate contains around 8% protein, 55% carbohydrate and 30% fat (most of which is saturated). Every 100g will deliver around 520kcal of energy, approximately 23mg of cholesterol, 220mg of calcium, 1.5mg of iron and 50mg of magnesium. It also contains a range of vitamins but does not contain any vitamin C. Chocolate contains serotonin and phenylethalamine, both of which help against mood swings and are mildly addictive. It also contains theobromine, which will result in cravings, so take care!

Q What is it about Coke that is so bad for my child's teeth?

A Coke contains two main ingredients which impact on teeth. The first is sugar and coke has loads of that and secondly it contains a substance called metaphosphoric acid which destroys the enamel. Discourage your child from drinking such drinks and encourage the consumption of water or sugar free squash type drinks.

Q What are the energy needs for adolescent boys and how do they differ from adolescent girls?

A Adolescent boys require something like 2,500–3,000kcal per day, which is in the order of 30% more than girls do. Those who are very actively engaged in sports are likely to need the upper end of these figures.

Q Why is calcium so important for young girls?

A Inadequate calcium intake is a common concern, especially for teenage girls, because lack of calcium at this time can significantly affect the development of osteoporosis (weak bones) later in life. It's not uncommon for teenagers to reduce or even stop drinking milk. In such cases yoghurt, cheese and perhaps even calcium-fortified drinks should be encouraged. Don't forget that bread is also a good source of calcium.

Q I know of a person who is unable to drink milk. Could you tell me why?

A Most of the world's population stop making lactase after the age of five years. Lactase is

85

the enzyme needed to break down the milk sugar lactose. Milk or dairy products (all of which contain lactose) consumed by people deficient in lactase result in stomach pain and discomfort. The condition is called lactose intolerance, and people who suffer from it are often advised to drink calcium enriched soy milk instead. If you think your child is suffering from this then speak to your health visitor or GP.

Q Why is it that obese or over-weight people can eat what I eat, which I don't think is excessive, but still do not lose weight?

A There may be a number of reasons, including the following:

● Over-weight people are covered with more fat, so they require less energy to keep them warm.

● When a person becomes obese or over-weight, they got there because of consuming too much food, too much of the wrong types of foods and probably were not active enough. Simply cutting back slightly may not be enough to lose weight, especially if their levels of physical activity do not increase. At this level of food reduction, they may simply stop putting weight on. To lose weight they will need to reduce the level of food even further and do this along with increased activity.

● Some illnesses can lead to obesity or weight gain, e.g. an under-active thyroid (hypothyroidism).

Q What is the best way to stop my young son eating crisps while watching television?

A Don't have them in the house. If you do not buy crisps (and other foods that do not contribute to good health), they would not be available to your child. If your son likes to snack, then encourage health-promoting foods like fruit, low-fat yoghurts or fromage frais.

Q If you were asked what, in one sentence, should be the main aim of our diets, what would you say?

A Our diets should promote optimum health.

Q How would you best advise an over-weight child to start exercising?

A For obese people, exercise should be started slowly and increased in intensity very gradually. Initial activities could include, for example, normal daily activities like walking. In time and depending on weight loss and level of fitness, they may be able to engage in something a little more strenuous, and moderate activity for 30–40 minutes a day perhaps 3–5 days per week should be encouraged. Before starting on any programme of physical activity, it is a good idea to discuss the options with a qualified expert and that includes your GP.

Q What is meant by Coeliac Disease?

A Coeliac Disease is a digestive disease that damages the small intestines and interferes with the absorption of nutrients. People who suffer from this problem are unable to tolerate a protein found in cereal products called gluten. Gluten is found in all products made from wheat, rye, barley and oats (though some sufferers can tolerate oats), so people suffering from the disease must avoid these foods.

Q You spoke earlier in your presentation of something called homocysteine and you spoke of it as a risk factor for heart disease. Could you give a little more detail please?

A Homocysteine is produced when the body breaks down protein, specifically when the body breaks down the essential amino acid called methionine. Under normal conditions the homocysteine is removed from the body or converted back to methionine, but a deficiency of B vitamins can lead to levels of homocysteine increasing. High levels of homocysteine in the blood damage the cells which line blood vessels allowing cholesterol to do its damage. That is why it's a risk factor associated with coronary heart disease.

Q Is there anything we can do to reduce the levels of homocysteine in our blood?

A Yes, the vitamins involved in controlling the levels of homocysteine are B6, B12 and especially folic acid. If your diet does not contain green leafy vegetables then you should consider taking a good multi-vitamin supplement.

Q What are best sources of dietary fibre?

A Dietary fibre is only to be found in foods of plant origin, not in meat. Fruit, vegetables, baked beans and unrefined cereal grains are excellent sources.

Q I understand that high levels of salt can result in high blood pressure, but what level is recommended that we can consume safely?

A It's generally agreed that we typically consume twice the salt we should be consuming. Try to keep to an intake of no more than 6g per day, and that means limit the amount of salt added to foods. In particular, read food labels; you may be very surprised by the number of canned or other processed foods that are high in salt.

Q I have recently heard the term 'ketogenic diet'. What is it?

A Ketogenic diets are diets that allow low levels of carbohydrate in the diet. As a result levels of fat are higher than they would normally be. Ketogenic diets are said to promote fat

87

breakdown in the body, and therefore are proposed to be the answer to fat loss (by some!). As fat is broken down, ketones are produced and these are smelly substances which can be smelt on the breath. Ketogenic diets are often used by elite bodybuilders prior to competition, where fat loss and increased muscle definition is the short-term aim. I have spoken to many such people who tell me that this type of diet works in the short term, but such diets do not promote health and are not sustainable. Ketogenic diets are sometimes promoted to people suffering from epilepsy, in conjunction with their medication. This should only be undertaken under the care of a paediatric dietitian.

Q What is hypoglycaemia?

A Hypoglycaemia is a very serious condition where levels of glucose in the blood fall to very low levels. The condition may occur if a diabetic patient eats too little, exercises too much, drinks alcohol without consuming enough carbohydrates or does not prepare or inject insulin properly. Signs of hypoglycaemia include weakness, sweating, confusion, heart palpitations and in severe cases coma or death.

Q Could you briefly explain what roles calcium plays in our body?

A Calcium is an essential mineral which makes up bones and teeth and is also crucial for the transmission of information along the nerves. Typically, women are much more often deficient in calcium than men, and the elderly, especially elderly women are particularly vulnerable to lack of calcium. Deficiency contributes to brittle bones (osteoporosis), gum disease and muscle cramps.

Q What are the sources of calcium?

A Milk and dairy products are good sources, but it can also be derived from calcium-fortified or enriched foods like breakfast cereals. Bread is also a good source.

Q I've heard that coffee reduces iron absorption. Is this true?

A Yes, drinking coffee within an hour of a meal can reduce iron absorption by up to 80%. This is a good reason not to drink coffee at breakfast, if your main source of dietary iron is breakfast cereals.

Q What are the best foods for controlling hunger?

A Those that are broken down slowly in the body, such as carbohydrates with a low GI, are excellent. Fresh fruit and vegetables are really good because of the fibre they contain. High fibre foods tend to make you feel fuller. Stay away from highly processed foods.

Q What is the best way to prevent children becoming over-weight?

A There are a number of things to consider. Most children tend to copy the eating habits of their parents, so set an example. Encourage your children to get interested in foods and their diet. Don't give children sweets, chocolate or crisps as a reward; they are treats only. Get them active, play with them. Children today are significantly less active than they were several decades ago and this is a problem contributed to by sedentary pastimes like television and computer games. Basically, feed your children health-promoting foods and encourage them to get active or increase their activity.

APPENDIX 1

Estimated Average Energy Requirements of Children up to 18 years of age

Energy requirements for girls

Age (in years)	Energy requirement (kcal/day)
1–3	1165
4–6	1545
7–10	1740
11–14	1845
15–18	2110

Energy requirements for boys

Age (in years)	Energy requirement (kcal/day)
1–3	1165
4–6	1545
7–10	1740
11–14	1845
15–18	2110

Source: *Dietary Reference Values for Food Energy and Nutrients for the United Kingdom.* Report on Health and Social Subjects 41. Department of Health 1991.

APPENDIX 2

Body Mass Index and Waist to Hip Ratio

Not suitable for children under the age of 18 unless it's plotted on a BMI chart and needs interpretation by a healthcare professional because the amount of body fat changes with age and differs between boys and girls.

Body Mass Index

All you have to do is follow these steps:

1 Weigh your child in kilograms (not pounds and ounces).

2 Measure the height of your child in metres (not feet and inches).

3 Multiply the height by itself, e.g. if your child is 1.2 metres high then multiple 1.2 by 1.2 which gives 1.32, this represents the height in metres squared (m2).

4 Now simply divide the weight in kilos by the height in metres squared.

Less than 18.5 is underweight.

Between 18.5–24.9 is normal weight.

Between 25–29.9 is overweight and

Greater than 30 is obese.

Let's work through an example.

Child's weight	=	52.5 kilograms
Child's height	=	1.35 metres

Using the method outlined above, you will need to multiple the child's height by itself, so it will be 1.35 x 1.35 = 1.82. Simply divide this into the child's weight which is 52.5 kilograms. 52.5/1.82 = 28.85. Check this figure with the figures in the table above and you will see that in this example, the child is over-weight.

There is a problem with this method however; because it does not take into account the weight of muscle, so that for example (and I know this will not relate to children) a bodybuilder or an athletic person may have a body mass index greater than 30. This would classify them as obese but in fact they may carry very little fat. This is a good time to mention a very important point with regards to weight loss.

If our child is over-weight or obese and we recognise they need to lose weight, it is body fat they need to lose. This is a good reason to emphasise healthy eating and an increase in physical activity rather than strict low calorie dieting because, if muscle mass is lost, then weight control is made more difficult later.

Waist to Hip Ratio (suitable for older teenagers and adults)

If the ratio of your child's waist to hip measurement is more than 0.8 (female) or 0.95 (male) then your child is over-weight. To calculate waist to hip ratio, all you have to do is follow these steps.

1 Measure your child's waist at its narrowest.

2 Measure their hips at their widest.

3 Divide the waist measurement by the hip measurement.

Let's work through an example for a male child.

The waist measurement is 75cm.

The hip measurement is 80cm.

We divide the waist by the hip measurement (i.e. 75/80) which gives 0.94.

This is below 0.95 so his measurement would be regarded as healthy.

APPENDIX 3

Glycaemic index of selected foods

Examples of foods and drinks with a glycaemic index below 60

Food	Glycaemic Index
All Bran	30
Apple juice	40
Apple muffin	44
Apricot	57
Baked beans	48
Banana	52
Basmati rice	58
Boiled potato	56
Broccoli	<15
Brown bread	58
Brown rice	55
Brussels sprouts	<15
Butter beans	36
Cabbage	<15
Capellini pasta	45
Carrot juice	45
Carrots	49
Celery	<15
Cherries	22
Chocolate (white)	44
Chocolate mousse	31
Corn chips (plain)	42
Cranberry juice	56
Crisps	54
Cucumber	<15
Custard	43
Digestive biscuits	58
Dried apple	29
Dried apricot	31
Fettuccine pasta	32

Food	Glycaemic Index
French beans	<15
Fresh apple	38
Fresh peach	28
Fresh pear	38
Fresh plums	39
Fructose	23
Grapefruit juice	48
Grapefruit	25
Grapes	52
Kidney beans (boiled)	29
Kiwi Fruit	55
Lactose	46
Lentils	29
Low-fat ice-cream	50
Low-fat yoghurt	33
Macaroni	45
Mango	51
Meat-filled ravioli	39
Muesli	56
Mushrooms	<15
Oat bran	55
Oatmeal cookie	55
Orange juice	52
Oranges	44
Pastry	59
Peanuts	<15
Peas	51
Peppers	<15
Pineapple juice	46
Plums	39

Food	Glycaemic Index
Popcorn	55
Porridge (non-instant)	49
Potato crisps	54
Pound cake	54
Prunes (pitted)	29
Quaker Oats	50
Raw cherries	22
Shredded Wheat	58
Skimmed milk	32
Soy beans (boiled)	16
Soya milk	30
Spaghetti (durum wheat)	55
Spaghetti (white)	38
Spaghetti (wholemeal)	37
Spinach	<15
Sucrose	59
Sweet corn	55
Tinned fruit cocktail	55
Tinned lentil soup	44
Tinned peaches	47
Tinned pears	44
Tomato soup	38
Tomatoes	15
Turnips	<15
Twix	44
Watercress	<15
Whole grain bread	46
Whole milk	27
Wholewheat spaghetti	37
Yam	51

Examples of foods and drinks with a glycaemic index above 60

Food	Glycaemic Index	Food	Glycaemic Index	Food	Glycaemic Index
Angel cake	67	Fruit flavour low-fat yoghurt	33	Shredded Wheat	69
Baked potato	85	Glucose	100	Special K	66
Bagel	72	Gluten-free bread	90	Steamed potato	65
Beetroot	64	Honey	87	Swede	72
Boiled new potato	70	Ice cream	61	Tinned apricots in syrup	64
Broad beans	79	Mashed potato	70	Wafer biscuits	77
Cheerios	74	Melon	65	Waffles	76
Cooked parsnips	97	Microwaved potato	82	Watermelon	72
Cornflakes	83	Pineapple	66	Weetabix	77
Croissant	67	Puffed Wheat	74	White bread	71
Doughnut	76	Raisins	64	White rice	72
French baguette	95	Ryvita	67	White rolls	73
Fresh new potatoes	62	Shortbread	64	Wholemeal bread	69
Fried potato (chips)	75				

As with all foods, the glycaemic index of potatoes is affected by a number of factors including the degree of processing (e.g. cooking times and temperatures) and the addition of other foods (e.g. butter). Having said that, it is not a good idea to add large amounts of butter to mashed potatoes simply to decrease the GI value. Remember butter is a saturated fat (not a good fat!) and its addition also increases the calorie content per serving.

APPENDIX 4

Summary of Nutritional Tips

● Fresh fruit and vegetables (5-a-day) are very important; these foods will supply important vitamins, minerals and fibre.

● Encourage children to participate in the planning and preparation of meals; this will emphasise the importance of the food they consume.

● Limit refined foods as much as possible, for example, brown bread is better than white bread.

● As a general rule encourage the consumption of fresh foods with as little processing as possible because processing removes important nutrients and fibre.

● Reduce the consumption of high-fat, high-sugar foods, e.g. cakes and biscuits etc. These foods are loaded with calories which contribute to obesity and poor health.

● Limit salt addition to food during cooking and also when on the plate. Excess salt contributes to high blood pressure.

● Do not force-feed; children are usually a good judge of how much they need to eat. It's better to give smaller portions and if the child wants more let them ask for more.

● Do not encourage dieting, but encourage healthy eating. A banana is better than a bar of chocolate and often it's less expensive.

● Encourage regular exercise/physical activity; lack of exercise is a major problem of all age groups, including children and is a contributor to obesity and heart disease.

● Discourage too much television and computer games; these often take the place of exercise, leading to problems later in life.

● Reduce consumption of high-sugar gassy drinks, substitute with fruit drinks. Sugar-free squashes are OK, but take care with artificial colours and flavours, as these may cause hyperactivity.

● Encourage the drinking of water, this with the higher intake of fibre (e.g. from fruit) and regular exercise will promote regular bowel movement, important for a healthy gut.

- Limit foods such as crisps, chips, pies, pasties, chocolate and sweets. High levels of fatty foods lead to obesity and high cholesterol; both are risk factors for heart disease. High levels of sugary foods lead to obesity and tooth decay and increase the risk of diabetes.

- Try grilling in place of frying, but if you must fry food, keep the fat to a minimum and change the oil often.

- Always ensure your child/children eat breakfast – porridge with a glass of orange juice is a great start to the day.

- Let's not be tempted to purchase foods we commonly refer to as 'junk' foods, e.g. crisps. If our children cannot see these foods in the home they are less likely to ask for them.

- We should try to purchase foods with simple ingredients and avoid foods containing salt, monosodium glutamate and artificial colours and flavours. Whole foods that are not processed or refined are more health-promoting than highly refined or processed foods.

- Keep cooking times to a minimum as cooking reduces the levels of vitamins in foods. Try steaming instead, in this way cooking times will be reduced.

- The best way to encourage our children to eat healthily and make a change in lifestyle is to lead by example, so let's do it with them.

APPENDIX 5

Smoothie Recipes

Banana Smoothie

Ingredients

2 Bananas

1 small pot Low-Fat Natural Yoghurt

$1/4$ litre Pineapple Juice

5–10 Ice cubes

Strawberry/Raspberry Smoothie

Ingredients

1 Small Punnet Strawberries

1 Small Punnet Raspberries

1 small pot Low-Fat Natural Yoghurt

$1/4$ litre Orange Juice

5–10 Ice cubes

Method

1. Chop the fruit into small pieces and place into a liquidizer.

2. Add the yoghurt and the fruit juice.

3. Mix for approximately 20–30 seconds (just long enough to produce a thick liquid).

4. Add the ice and mix to a smooth liquid (approximately 30 seconds).

NB Note that no sugar is added to the recipe; there is enough sugar in the fruit. Any fruit can be used. Use the same basic recipe but simply change the fruit. I have found that blackberries combined with blackcurrants make a great smoothie.

APPENDIX 6

Examples of good snacking foods

An apple

Dried apricots

Milk or milk shake

Smoothie

2 oatmeal cookies

An orange

A banana

Whole grain sandwich

Bowl of porridge

Fromage frais or low-fat yoghurt

Vegetables

Hummus

Baked beans on toast

Celery sticks stuffed with cottage or grated cheese

Hard-boiled eggs

Home made oatcakes

Egg baked in a ramekin

APPENDIX 7

Reference Nutrient Intakes for Selected Vitamins and Minerals

Vitamins	Young Children			Males			Females		
Age in years	1–3	4–6	7–10	11–14	15–18	19–50	11–14	15–18	19–50
Thiamin (mg per day)	0.5	0.7	0.7	0.9	1.1	1.0	0.7	0.8	0.8
Riboflavin (mg per day	0.6	0.8	1.0	1.2	1.3	1.3	1.1	1.1	1.1
Niacin (mg per day)	8.0	11.0	12.0	15.0	18.0	17.0	12.0	14.0	13.0
Vitamin B6 (mg per day)	0.7	0.9	1.0	1.2	1.5	1.4	1.0	1.2	1.2
Vitamin B12 (µg per day)	0.5	0.8	1.0	1.2	1.5	1.5	1.2	1.5	1.5
Folic Acid (µg per day)	70	100	150	200	200	200	200	200	200
Vitamin C (mg per day)	30.0	30.0	30.0	35.0	40.0	40.0	35.0	40.0	40.0
Vitamin A (µg per day)	400	400	500	600	700	700	600	600	600
Vitamin D (µg per day)	7.0	–	–	–	–	–	–	–	–

Minerals	Young Children			Males			Females		
Age in years	1–3	4–6	7–10	11–14	15–18	19–50	11–14	15–18	19–50
Calcium (mg per day)	350	450	550	1000	1000	700	800	800	700
Iron (mg per day)	6.9	6.1	8.7	11.3	11.3	8.7	14.8	14.8	14.8
Magnesium (mg per day)	85	120	200	280	300	300	280	300	270
Zinc (mg per day)	5.0	6.5	7.0	9.0	9.5	9.5	9.0	7.0	7.0
Copper (mg per day)	0.4	0.6	0.7	0.8	1.0	1.2	0.8	1.0	1.2
Selenium (µg per day)	15	20	30	45	70	75	60	60	60
Sodium (mg per day)	500	700	1200	1600	1600	1600	1600	1600	1600

mg   milligrams or one-thousandth of a gram

µg   micrograms or one-millionth of a gram

APPENDIX 8

Reference Nutrient Intake for Protein (grams per day)

Age	Boys	Girls
0–3 months	12.5	
4–6 months	12.7	
7–9 months	13.7	
10–12 months	14.9	
1–3 years	14.5	
4–6 years	19.7	
7–10 years	28.3	
11–14 years	42.1	41.2
15–18 years	55.2	45.0

Source: *Dietary Reference Values for Food Energy and Nutrients for the United Kingdom.* Report on Health and Social Subjects 41. Department of Health 1991.

Examples

1. 55g portion of chicken breast would give approximately 11g of protein.
2. A tablespoon full of baked beans would give approximately 3g of protein.
3. 45g serving of porridge with 320ml of skimmed milk would give approximately 15g of protein.